Healing Presence

The Essence of Nursing

JOELLEN GOERTZ KOERNER, RN, PhD, FAAN, and founder of NurseMetriX, is an author, editor, speaker, researcher, educator, and nurse executive leader of international renown. She is the past president of the American Organization of Nurse Executives (AONE) and 2005 recipient of the Lifetime Achievement Award from the AONE Institute for Patient Care Research and Education. With extensive executive-level management and leadership experience in health care administration, education, regulation, and e-commerce, her initial career efforts focused on nursing education and service in corporate health systems. She then worked in virtual education with curriculum modeling and delivery at the intersection of the philosophy and practice of professional nursing.

As founder of NurseMetriX, Dr. Koerner designed applications of corporate, scientific, and information technology for Web-based innovations in the nursing profession. Her international and voluntary work is focused on workforce development for underrepresented sectors of society.

Healing Presence

The Essence of Nursing

JoEllen Goertz Koerner, RN, PhD, FAAN

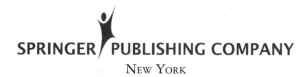

SPRINGER PUBLISHING COMPANY
NEW YORK

Springer Publishing Company, LLC
11 West 42nd Street
New York, NY 10036
www.springerpub.com

Acquisitions Editor: Sally J. Barhydt
Production Editor: Carol Cain
Cover design: Mimi Flow
Covert Art: David Stirts
Composition by Apex Publishing, LLC

07   08   09   10/   5   4   3   2   1

Library of Congress Cataloging-in-Publication Data

Koerner, JoEllen Goertz.
 Healing presence : the essence of nursing / JoEllen Goertz Koerner.
  p. ; cm.
 Includes bibliographical references and index.
 ISBN-13: 978-0-8261-1575-1 (alk. paper)
 ISBN-10: 0-8261-1575-6 (alk. paper)
 1. Nursing—Psychological aspects.   2. Healing—Psychological aspects.   3. Holistic nursing.   4. Nurse and patient.   I. Title.
 [DNLM: 1. Nursing Care—methods.   2. Mind-Body and Relaxation Techniques—nursing.   WY 100 K78h 2007]

RT86.K6448 2007
610.73—dc22   2007005727

Printed in the United States of America by Bang Printing.

This book is dedicated to the Universal Spirit that unites and heals us all.

Contents

Preface

AN INVITATION

Through a long and rewarding career in nursing I have been privileged to support and learn from many about the wellness-illness patterns that mark the human experience. It is frequently an illness event that slows us down, inviting us to step outside normal routines to reevaluate the beliefs and patterns that create the life we live. Cares of the day become insignificant when one is confronted with one's mortality. The focus shifts to the deeper questions of the soul.

Occasionally when we are ill, we are fortunate enough to have the support and safety of a caring relationship in which we can ponder with vulnerability and reflect with candor on our fundamental beliefs, our assumptions and expectations for ourselves and others. We begin to sort through the panorama of lived experiences we have encountered and discern how we have used them to understand and ascribe meaning to life as a whole and to our life specifically.

Nursing education taught me skills in assessment and intervention to relieve suffering and promote healing of the body. Experiences as a middle child helped me develop a deep intuition about what was central to the issue at hand when viewpoints varied. The resulting capacity of managing subtly by hearing behind the words and seeing beneath the action helped facilitate clarity for myself and others. However, later in my career, as I was caring for my daughter in her near-death experience, she taught me a deeper and richer way of being with people. From her I truly came to understand what creates a healing environment for people faced with a health crisis, and we both became more in the exchange.

It is humbling to realize how little our external efforts impact healing. True healing versus physical curing arises from an internal mechanism residing within the soul of each of us. This innate capacity is enhanced when recognized and honored by one who offers a healing presence in the caring experience. Many individuals from all walks of life have served as witness and support for someone suffering, facilitating that healing force within their loved one. So it is with profound respect for the power of love to heal that I have created this book on healing presence.

Nursing is at the crossroads, facing shortages of unparalleled proportion at a time when society is experiencing health care challenges of great magnitude. As older nurses retire, the next generation is nowhere evident. The nursing profession has spent so much effort in the recent past to attain scientific legitimacy within the health care industry that the core essence of the discipline has been misplaced. At the *center* of professional nursing lies the authentic presence of the nurse, the intent and commitment that brings the nurse to the profession in the first place. When there is congruence between who they are and what they do, nurses bring their souls to work. This balance is experienced as a healing presence that potentiates the patient's self-healing capacity. Both the nurse and patient experience meaning in their exchange and each becomes more whole.

This book is designed to place twenty-first-century nursing into a timeless paradigm, one that transcends the economic, political, and technological culture of the day. It is important to remember that nursing is a social mandate and has been part of the communal fabric since the dawning of civilization. Birth, death, and health-illness are a part of the legacy of humankind, which requires the assistance of others. Exciting developments in science and technology have made the role of the nurse richer and more complex. We now have an array of tools and services to offer those we care for that were not possible for our predecessors. But the unifying, underlying essence of our work is the timeless and profound healing presence we offer that enhances the exploration and creation of meaning in the inevitable health challenges faced by individuals, families, and groups whose lives we are privileged to touch.

This offering is a compilation of information and insights accrued as I traversed a professional journey. In the early stages of my chosen vocation, I quickly discovered that nursing is truly an art as well as a science; information needed interpretation for appropriate application. My interests in both were met with another realization that, at its core, nursing called for something more. It required an exchange of the human spirit.

Through the years, my study became increasingly focused on the emerging fields of quantum science, philosophy, and metaphysics. In that juncture of body-mind-spirit a synthesis of wholeness was finally grasped. The underlying philosophy expressed in this book reflects an appreciation of, and a place for, all aspects of life and human endeavor. Because life is so big, and the world becoming increasingly small, the beliefs and values of all we serve in nursing are asking to be recognized, respected, and honored in our awareness and our healing work.

Although theories come and go in just a few centuries or even decades, inklings of the mystical are found in the writings of great personalities the world over. People like Einstein, William Blake, and Carl Jung have modeled that deep thought is always inspired from within. Their reflections are woven throughout the scientific exploration undertaken here as an effort to interweave the philosophical and spiritual into our predominant frame of reference.

Growing up in a small rural community of 1,000 people, I discovered the power of the written word. I quickly learned that through a book one could engage in an inner dialogue with people across time and distance. This book is not meant to be a comprehensive scientific review, but rather an introduction to conversations with some of the finest minds in existence. It is a small effort to introduce you to my friends (as noted in the many references inviting you to join their dialogue). It is an invitation to remember your call to nursing, to reengage with the passion and commitment that inspired you. It is a statement of gratitude for all you have contributed to the life of humankind in general, and mine in particular. It is a celebration of the power of the human spirit that is manifest everywhere we practice. And it is a statement of gratitude to All-That-Is for the privilege of sharing the life journey with so many at this time in history.

> *Ask that I may be forgiven if my pen*
> *has gone astray or my foot has slipped,*
> *for to plunge into the abyss of the Divine*
> *Mysteries is a perilous thing and no easy*
> *task is it to seek to discover the Unclouded*
> *Glory which lies behind the veil.*
>
> Al-Ghazali

JoEllen Goertz Koerner

Foreword

REFLECTIONS OF A NURSE HEALER

...and at the end of all our exploring will be to arrive where we started ... and to know the place for the first time.

T. S. Eliot
Little Gidding

All nurses, regardless of our career paths, have at one time or another enjoyed the privilege of sharing our healing presence with patients. This opportunity to contribute to the patient's health and well-being using compassion and empathy has been what most nurses would say drew them into the profession. This call to our work, acknowledged as timeless, has not really had the center stage it might, given its magnetic pull to the profession. As a matter of fact, in my 35 years as a nurse I have seen the topic of nursing's essence discussed more when the profession was near a drought either in recruits or in role satisfaction. Our cyclical conversations have been inadequate for such an important cornerstone of nursing's work. It seems the energy so needed to fuel the profession lies deep in this aspect of our work. How we can collectively learn to more effectively use it is key.

Drilling Down to the Essence

I have often viewed and described the work of nursing in two dimensions, doing and being. All nurses understand the doing dimension of nursing. So much of a nurse's preparation, socialization, and role definition lies in what nurses do. The doing skills and technical accountabilities are what keep nurses running and very busy. This dimension of nursing's work has clearly changed, grown, and become more complex over time. Doing is clearly more concrete, measurable, and generally what has been perceived to be the valued aspect.

The being dimension of the role of nurse is less about what nurses do and more about the how. The focus of being and how the nurse comes to the bedside receives less time in a nurse's preparation, socialization, and even role definition. Admittedly, this being dimension is more difficult to describe, harder to measure, and although valued by nurses and those patients who benefit from it, has not always been at the center of what is rewarded. Being is what slows down the nurse so that space is created for an authentic, deep connection with the patient and healing. The work of being has remained constant over time. Embedded in the being dimension of the role lies the essence of nursing, and it is here that the call to the profession is actualized.

One might say that over my career I have had a preoccupation and conversation around the essence of nursing. When years have passed since I have seen certain colleagues and we end up in conversation about nursing, I am certain they say, "she's still at it." I even bore myself at times. Nevertheless, bringing focus and language to this being dimension has been my lifelong work.

Ten years into my nursing career while in graduate school I fell deeply into the study of the humanistic psychologists, particularly Carl Rogers. His theories and writings, *On Becoming a Person,* and *Person Centered Approach,* brought me a new perspective on the being aspect of my bedside practice. The biggest shift was looking inward at myself first before looking at how I might be more effective in working with others. Rogers's delineation of the conditions necessary for this deep connection with patients gave me a loom into which to weave the threads of my work about being. These conditions of genuineness, acceptance, and empathetic understanding were fitting for the preparation of coming to the bedside to be fully present for the patient. One might even say that for nurses these conditions are obligatory in occupying the space for healing with patients.

As nurses we have been taught and have learned a fair amount about the importance of empathy. We have witnessed its effect on patients and learned from our experiences, and nurses have earned well-deserved credibility in its delivery. We have spent little time, however, on our individual development of genuineness and acceptance. It is as if once we have received the call into nursing these two other qualities were assumed to be in place. Nurses, as great as we might be in the eyes of those we serve, are as human as anyone. As such, we come with our own individual work to do as we journey toward our potential. Seated so close to the patient in the practice of nursing, this individual obligation takes on crucial importance.

The condition of being genuine in our relationships with patients and others seems welcoming. What an invitation to be who I am, which is not as simple at times as it may seem. Besides acknowledging our humanness, being genuine implies a deep awareness and knowledge of self. Moreover, it calls for an appreciation of self with all the beauty and bruises that our true self reflects. The acceptance of our self as imperfect creates the capacity to be more open, transparent, and vulnerable. This authenticity plays a key role in how we are seen and experienced by others. Being genuine is a necessary condition in order for others to be real with us.

I have found Rogers's second condition of acceptance dependent on the capacity to be genuine. When I am accepting of my true self, I am more accepting of others and where they are. Just as self-acceptance implies being free from preconceived notions about myself, accepting others requires the giving up of any bias or predetermined perceptions about where others should be. This means no prejudice, labels, or judging of others. It is only when we are fully accepting of our true selves that we are able to be fully open to accepting others. The gift of acceptance is the nurturant space it creates for others to discover more of their true selves.

One can easily see how development of a nurse's capacity for genuineness and acceptance influences the capacity for Rogers's third condition of empathetic understanding. The ability to understand and to feel the patient's journey, struggle, and emotions, as the patient experiences them, is the ultimate privilege of the role of nurse. This is not new territory for nurses. Capacity, however, will be enhanced, perhaps even transformed, with a deeper self-knowledge, acceptance, and new awareness.

This journey with self opens one's eyes to see new potential. We as nurses can well imagine the impact it could have in serving patients. Can we imagine at the same time the new potential and energy that would be created with renewed wholeness in nurses and nursing? The answer lies in our individual and collective willingness to claim, embrace, and become our essence . . . one nurse at a time.

Walk slowly with intent, courage and a sense of inquiry through the pages of wisdom that follow. JoEllen Koerner, one of nursing's most entrusted friends and healers, is our guide to discovery and coming home.

Julie MacDonald, RN, MSN
Chief Operating Officer
St. Joseph Mercy Healthcare System

SECTION I

Introduction

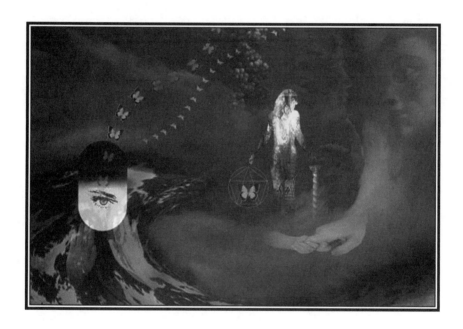

Fear not the strangeness that you feel.
the future must enter you
long before it happens.
Just wait for the birth,
for the hour of new clarity.

Rainer Maria Rilke

CHAPTER 1

Nursing

A Sacred Work

To possess the will that nurses our visions &
brings us closer to the path of angels,
that infuses us with compassion &
makes us glow like a soft amber—
that is the secret of wisdom.

Henryk Skolimowski

The profession of nursing is a tribe, complete with our own culture, customs, and mores. Early tribal groups found strength and flexibility through the differentiation of task and orientation as hunter-gatherers, artisans, and healers shared in caring for the needs of the community. So too, contemporary nursing is offered by practitioners with a bias for the rigors of science, the aesthetics of artistic expression, or the meaning of spiritual orientation. Individually and collectively our differences converge on a shared mission, the support of healing on this planet.

This book is an invitation to examine our world and our work from the multiple perspectives of our clan. Given the multifaceted nature of the topic and the tribe, this offering is comprised of various perspectives and interweaving themes. The voices and viewpoints are varied, creating a mosaic of models and metaphors that speak to our differing orientations to the role. Reflections and insights from colleagues give depth and meaning to our shared experience of caring.

This book is a composite of findings and innovations grouped into various orientations that may best fit your particular worldview. For the quintessential nurse scientist, the first section of this offering focuses on the unfolding discoveries of quantum physics and our understanding of health and illness from the new science perspective. Section II looks at health and healing through the lens of philosophy and spirituality, identifying new models for transpersonal caring. The final section of this book speaks to nursing practice from the perspective of beliefs and values, and the artistic cocreative activity of choice and action.

Feel free to wander through the rich tapestry woven from threads of insight given by so many courageous pioneers in the healing field. Add your own discoveries and wisdom as you reflect on your call to the profession, your experiences, your insights, and your aspirations. Share them with colleagues as we cocreate the context and the processes for our sacred and ever-unfolding work.

A RETURN OF THE FEMININE HEALING ENERGY

We are living in a most extraordinary and opportune time, as the world faces a crucial juncture in the history of humankind. While the last Renaissance focused on the merging of art and science, this current awakening includes the illumination of our personal philosophy, the embracing of our own wisdom. We are poised to come home; to embrace the essence of our own wholeness.

As we continue into the new millennium, some of us sense that this is a major turning point in the long human journey. As we perceive the difference between the superficial and the substantive, we recognize what is being born while surrounded by what is dying. To witness life at this level, we must view the process from soul territory. Fortunately, we are no strangers here. This is the very center of the nursing domain.

The epoch of nursing began with the inhalation of the first breath of humankind. It is a story of presence and support, defined by witness and engagement, guided by compassion and caring. Ours is a story filled with ethos, intrigue, breakthroughs and setbacks, moments of beauty and periods of darkness. It is a story of the feminine healing energy moving through the ages. This pattern forms a seed-crystal for the notion of watchfulness; the practice of seeing and being seen by the Source.

On the physical level our portals of observation include two eyes, two ears, two nostrils, and a mouth. Yet, inherent in the feminine healing energy is the subtle ability to *see fully with an "unseen eye"*—to take in the whole—with a compassionate, caring heart, and detached vision.

Paradoxically, the ever-expanding field of classical science focused on masculine qualities is couched in the oft unseen field of feminine energy, the most essential element in the healing journey. For those we are privileged to serve, we provide the "source of mercy that helps others untie their tangles" (Briskin, 2005). Such is the nature of the realm of *active receptivity,* the sacred essence of nursing.

Unlike Western society, other cultures honor the place of the feminine function in their stories. In Hindu legend, the Seven Rishi look and watch over the whole of the universe. Jewish tradition refers to the Seven Eyes of God looking out upon the world.

This way of seeing and being requires a specific responsibility for watching over things of the soul. Such a witness takes us deep into the farthest reaches of perception and consciousness. Seeing fully takes us to the essence of our higher selves, that which is our connection point to All-That-Is. From this portal we recognize that there is something we all know that deepens our identification with others and the very earth itself. We come alive with feeling, sensing the unbroken consciousness that creates a vibration of shared meaning that flows as an expression of heart, mind, and will. This is the space of *active receptivity.*

Such a place prompts an apprehension of wholeness, which is the receptive feminine function in the universe. Reb Zalman observed:

> The other thing that is necessary is to have women involved. Because it's in the nature of the masculine vision to see the figure and ignore the ground. In other words that which is erect and that which enters and that which has power, and that which deposits sperm, and that which is active, and so on and so forth. (Cited in Briskin, 2005, p. 9)

Too often there is an ignoring of those who receive, or contain, or hold. Much focus is placed on the object, leaving little awareness of the field in which it sets. One sees the black letters on the page without conscious recognition of the white space that surrounds them. Reb Zalman continues:

> I can't see the wind, but I see the flag in the wind.... Though I don't see the wind I see the flag moving. I understand that what I'm seeing is not just the flag, but it's flag and wind.... In similar fashion when I look at a river, it's the bed and it's the water. But river is the bed and the water together; it's the figure and ground together.

The active element of receptivity, this feminine function, fosters the construct of wholeness by making the object or event more than simply an interrelationship of parts. It is the active principle of wholeness, a figure-ground dynamic that exposes this invisible half, the one that gives context and meaning to that which it gently uplifts and holds. And in this undivided space, we are complete.

Many nursing actions take place against a background invisible to the eye not attuned to its subtle presence. To be truly conscious of the essence of the total experience is to continually seek the invisible half of wholeness. Here we uncover more information about what is transpiring within the dynamic nature of figure-ground relationship. For those who truly offer a healing presence, this awareness is the key to harmonizing the human with the spiritual. Theologian Paul Tillich describes God as the "ground of all being":

> If I want to see God, I'm trying to make a figure out of God. And that's what gets us in trouble. Because God cannot become a figure, always being ground.... But if we were to see as we are seen, as we are being created, as we are being made every moment, then everything is always in a field, and is connected with that field. (Cited in Briskin, 2005, p. 12)

As we revisit the archetypal feminine, it holds a very different image than is currently portrayed in contemporary society. From the Grail legends, Robert Sardello notes:

> The women of the Grail are representatives of the soul which houses qualities necessary for transforming the self, for realizing that true individuality lies in coming to know ourselves as human spiritual beings. None, absolutely none, of the women figures of the Grail are passive; they are all receptive, and a totally new, active sense of the quality of the feminine slowly dawns on the reader. (Quoted in Sussman, 1995, p. 173)

At this critical juncture for humanity, individuals are remembering the archetypal feminine qualities. This is fostering a new consciousness in the larger healing field. Both women and men are increasingly working with the feminine energies of cycle, rhythm, resonance, reciprocity and right relationship that interact directly with all things, including mother earth.

Accompanying this movement towards integral medicine is a spiritual revolution regarding what we can become as *human spiritual beings*. The qualities of the divine feminine are moving into a place of prominence as they renew us and the healing communities to which we belong. The essence of these feminine traits promotes an instinct for cooperation and an embracing of diversity in its many dynamic forms. At the same time, the inclusive language of the feminine offers hope and encouragement for an enhanced future.

Respect is the hallmark of this radically receptive field. Bordering on reverence, it is a simple personal respect for the patient, for colleagues, for the self. It is also an impersonal awareness at a deeper level, a sensing that we share space on a sacred healing journey with everything in the universe. *A Course in Miracles* states that "we heal a brother by recognizing his worth." As we witness for another, respecting and honoring what is observed can be the catalyst for transformation.

As the feminine energy is remembered, embraced and, once again, consciously used in integral medicine, the emerging wholeness is nothing less than profound. The balancing of the masculine and feminine is the transform-ing work that is birthing new world order. We are moving from an era guided by the Declaration of Independence, where models of autonomy and power reigned supreme. Unfolding discoveries in science and art continue to reveal a deeper theme of cooperation and cocreation running through every aspect of life. We have come to realize that each of us is the earth, the air, the sun, and a deeply connected part of one another. Thus, our emerging new worldview holds the promise of the birth of the Declaration of *Inter*dependence (Suzuki, 2002).

Worldview: Individual Perspective on How Life Works

Our interaction with all aspects of our world starts with how we view that world. Pessimistic eyes watch the undoing of our "old story" and feel despair when examining life from a partial, or limited viewpoint rather than seeing a larger picture. Cynical vision laced with judgment leads one to see evi-dence of imperfection. Soul-full eyes, however, see a larger, more holistic, and more realistic picture. These perceptive eyes penetrate the materialism and reductionism of our times, connecting historical patterns with new scientific evidence to gain insight into humanity's unfolding. From this vantage point one can see the larger context without overlooking the details of the present moment. This perspective facilitates tough optimism and practical expectancy within the chaotic unfolding of our times, fostering a sense of the optimistic hopefulness rather than despair and hopelessness.

Learning is our birthright; we are born with the innate ability to imagine, wonder, invent, and explore our way into unknown territory as we explore paradoxical and perplexing questions (Vaill, 1996). From our first breath we observe and sense, take things apart and put them back together again, wonder about the vastness of the universe and our place within it. The starting point of this awareness is awe and wonder. As much as we are an independent entity in the universe, we are also a partner with it. We are both thrilled and perplexed by our human condition. And in our irrepressible pursuit towards understanding, we create our world.

A sense of crisis is permeating our perceptions of the world. Many indi-viduals and large social institutions subscribe to an outdated worldview that is inadequate to deal with the larger issues of the day. New concepts in physics have shifted our understanding of the universe from the mechanistic and linear worldview of Descartes and Newton to the holistic and interconnected ecological view fostered by discoveries in quantum physics, cellular biology, and neuroscience. Advances in science and technology enable us to observe patterns and structures within the universe, giving us a new story of the natural world. Those unfamiliar with this new learning are limited in being able to fully see, integrate, and appreciate the story of unity and wholeness, reciprocity, interdependence, and cocreation within the unifying web of life (Capra, 1996).

Networks of order are emerging within the ecological, human, and technical worlds. Internally, a magnificently complex, pattern-seeking, living network of self-adjusting neurons connect our mind/brain. We are discovering that our thoughts have a powerful role in shaping our mind and brain, literally changing the physical structure of the brain. Human intelligence is not a fragmented and independent process, but rather a biological and social one. Meaning is constructed by matching new learning with existing patterns, creating new networks of internal and external connections.

Feelings and emotions are the guiding force for the holistic and networked process of active engagement underlying the construction of knowledge and meaning. Just as the mechanical model of the universe is being dismantled, so is the disconnected model of our mind-brain-body system (Marshall, 2005). As this awareness is shifting, so is our model for nursing practice.

Healing Presence: Ground, Field, and Witness

All health professions are being redefined as this new epoch unfolds. Nursing has traditionally been viewed as an art and a science. Our theories, curriculum, and practice models reflect this framework. Florence Nightingale observed that:

> Nursing is an art, and if it is to be made an art, it requires as exclusive a devotion, as hard a preparation as any painter's or sculptor's work; for what is the having to do with dead canvas or cold marble, compared to having to do with the living body, the temple of God's spirit. It is one of the Fine Arts; I had almost said the finest of the Fine Arts. (Calabria & Macrae, 1994, p. 183)

Careful examination on her reflection reveals yet a third dimension that underscores our profession, the context of *active receptivity,* which is the essence of a healing presence.

THE NURSING TRIAD: A MODEL FOR HEALING

As we come to understand the implicit third dimension of nursing we begin to comprehend the emergence of its three-fold framework: science, art, and essence. When all three domains are present in the nurse-person relationship, a healing gestalt occurs.

> *Science: Nurses are scientists*—Professional nursing is founded on a body of knowledge derived from science and research. Measured evidence forms a theoretical framework of the external physical world as the foundation, the object or focus of our clinical practice. This is the *evaluator aspect* of nursing, which comes from the *realm of concrete thought*. Facts, data, and logic guide our practice through evidence-based protocols and standards, which point our observations and choices towards predetermined outcomes.
>
> *Art: Nurses are artists*—Experience-based mastery leads to subtle pattern recognition from multiple perspectives, the field or ground of our practice. This *interpreter aspect* of nursing is from the *realm of abstract thought*. Intuition and active awareness of the understated fosters discernment and pattern recognition, which then guides synthesis of unrelated parts into a larger whole. Individualized personal care that supports the interior world of the patient is thus created.
>
> *Essence: Nurses are a healing presence*—An authentic and patient presence creates a space of *active receptivity* for the person (and their family) that potentiates their own inner resources. The feminine healing function of the *witness aspect* of nursing comes from the *realm of no-mind—pure consciousness*. Guided by the intent to support what is in the highest good for the person and family, we create an empty space of open expectancy, which allows individuals to connect with their inner wisdom and innate power to heal. As we trust in the other to grow and in ourselves to care, we have the courage to go into the unknown together.

Because there is simultaneous attention to the exterior world, the inner world, and the unmanifest now, the soul is also invited to participate. When we include the numinous in our shared space, transformative insight and energy emerge, enlarging the experience for both. And in that shared exchange, each becomes more. Carl Rogers observed that, "The degree to which I can create relationships which facilitate the growth of others as separate persons is a measure of the growth I have achieved in myself."

Nurses bring science, art, and essence to the individual and family, nursing is the heart and soul, the primary surveillance system, for the health of society. Because of this fact, a crisis of major proportion is imminent. While political, economic, and environmental issues challenge society, the increasing global shortage of nurses offers one of the greatest hazards to the health and well-being of humankind.

Medical practices vary in different parts of the world, depending on the tools and healing models of the culture. Nursing, on the other hand, is a universal phenomenon. Daily, and nightly, in every part of the world, millions of nurses stand alongside people in need, helping them with maintenance of activities of daily living such as mobility, elimination, and pain management. Nurses also assist the well in maintaining their health status through educating the public about adequate nutrition and exercise as well as the power of good mental health practices. Finally, and most importantly, nurses also accompany people in their journey towards a peaceful death, supporting families and loved ones in the process. Helping individuals, families, and society manage their inevitable health challenges, while finding meaning in the illness event, is at the core of what it means to be a nurse.

Nursing, as a global community, is in a unique position as midwife to help birth the "new story" for humanity. For this we have been preparing. For this we must utilize all the knowledge available to creatively practice the science, art, and essence of nursing.

Science: The Foundation of Knowledge, Which Guides Our Practice

Today we stand on the threshold of a revolution as daring as Einstein's discovery of relativity. On the frontier of science new ideas are emerging that challenge everything we have come to believe about the world and how it works. Discoveries are being made that demonstrate what philosophies and religions have held as true: humanity is more extraordinary than a mere physical machine that lives in a self-determined world. Through a dynamic quantum field we are ever-changing and deeply connected to *all that is.*

Scientists in various disciplines have been carrying out well-designed experiments whose results transcend the beliefs of current biology and physics. At core, what they have uncovered is the fact that we are not a collection of chemical reactions, but rather, an energetic charge. All living things are a coalescence of energy emerging from a universal, pulsating energy field connected to every other thing in the universe. This potent field is responsible for the highest functions of our mind. As an information source it guides the growth and development of our bodies. It influences our brain, our heart, and our memory. As radical as it may seem, this field, called the universal zero point field, rather than genes or germs, determines whether we are healthy or ill. It is, in the end, the force that must be tapped in order to heal (McTaggart, 2002).

Conventional science is grounded in the idea that matter is the building block of all things. Life, mind, and awareness are held to be secondary phenomena of matter. In the prevailing science, elementary particles make atoms, atoms make molecules, molecules make cells including neurons, neurons make the brain, and the brain makes awareness. The theory of causation holds that the interactions between the elementary particles create various forms of matter, moving from smaller to larger objects in predictable fashion. Dualistic either-or and cause-effect thinking have been the hallmark of reason for more than 400 years.

Quantum physics uncovers a reality more dynamic and connected than that put forward by conventional science. Upon examining this evolving research, one learns that several discoveries have already determined that rather than a universe of static certainty, matter at the most fundamental level, and the world that it builds, is uncertain and unpredictable, a state of pure potential and infinite possibility (Gleck, 1987). Subatomic particles are not seen as solid objects, but rather as vibrating and indeterminate packets of energy that cannot be precisely quantified or controlled. These energy packets can take on the quality of a particle, and either stay confined in a small space, spread over a large region of space-time in wavelike fashion, or do both simultaneously, that is, test out all possible new electron orbits at once.

Werner Heisenberg, an architect of quantum theory, established the Uncertainty Principle, which demonstrates that nothing is certain: there are no definite locations for these quantum energy packets, only a likelihood, a probability that they may settle into a specified pattern. Based upon this finding, cause-and-effect relationships no longer exist at the subatomic level, for stable-looking atoms suddenly elect to transfer from one energy state to another in an unpredictable leap (Heisenberg, 1971). Suddenly, amidst the known and expected, we are aware of the startling and unpredictable quantum-leap activity surrounding us. An unsettling quickening of activity and possibility is now the new hallmark of our times.

Quantum physics demonstrates that subatomic particles have a capacity for cooperation. They not only get in synch, they are also highly interlinked by bands of common electromagnetic fields so they can communicate with each other, like multiple tuning forks resonating together. As they get into phase together, they begin to act like one giant subatomic particle, creating a single large wave. What is done to one then affects the whole. Coherence establishes communication and high levels of quantum order (Bohm & Hiley, 1993).

Traditional science defines relationship by geographic proximity. Now the concept of nonlocality shatters this foundational principle of conventional physics. Once in contact with another, a quantum entity such as an electron retains a connection even when separated by time and space. Actions of one will continue to influence the actions of the other, no matter how far they are separated by time or distance (Nadeau & Kafatos, 2002). This phenomenon explains the power of prayer and meaningful relationships in the healing experience.

One of the most essential ingredients of this interconnected universal web of energy is the impact on the awareness of the person observing it. In classic physics, an experimenter is considered separate and apart from the experiment. The scientist is simply an impartial observer in the process. In contrast, quantum physics reveals that the state of all possibility is collapsed into a set entity when it is observed or measured. There is a strong relationship between the observer and the observed. In fact, the observer creates the observed object (Pribram, 1991). In other words, nothing in the world exists as an actual *thing* outside of our observing it, so, every minute of the day we create our world.

Classic laws of science have been very useful for describing fundamental properties of motion such as locomotion and respiration, and for explaining how basic body processes such as digestion and sensory input operate. But classic physics and biology have been unable to explain fundamental issues such as how we think, why arms and legs develop differently, how cells cure themselves of cancer, and how we know what we know. The emerging model of science begins to uncover a deeper reality, one that more fully explains the mysteries of the universe and our place within it. Implications of the new science for nursing practice will be explored in Section II.

Art: The Intuitive Skill of Clinical Reasoning

Both art and science are unique forms of language describing the same reality, with art leading the way. Artists and authors, especially those writing science fiction, depict what is about to be born in society. Art begins with a vision. It is preverbal in nature and precedes abstract ideas as well as the words and actions that describe and explore them. Visionary artists (nurses) alert others that a shift is about to occur because their vision is a particular prescience. They mysteriously incorporate into their work features of a physical description that science later discovers or proves (Shlain, 1991).

Nurses walk between two worlds, the concrete world of a scientist and the abstract world of an artist. Our craft depends on a well-developed sense of aesthetics: if it does not look right, it is not functioning properly. The intuitive capacity of the nurse is the heart of the sentinel function at the bedside, which notes a subtle shift heralding a potential crisis. Early identification assures intervention with the least amount of effort to restore balance.

Physicians most trust the nurse who lives in the realm of the aesthetic subtle. This nurse will call and report, "All vital signs are normal, but something is wrong; come now!" This nurse is sensing a faint shift in pattern that lies below the surface of articulation or measurement. Intuition and an appreciation for symmetry are guardians in the understated background of surveillance. Well developed, they are the gift a master practitioner brings to her or his profession.

Nurses rely heavily on the intuitive visual-spatial right hemisphere of their brain. At the same time, scientific rigor builds a deep repository of facts and data that figure into the logic and reason emanating from the left hemisphere. As scientists, they break the nature of things into discrete parts to analyze their relationships in reductionistic fashion. As artists, nurses synthesize varying aspects of the person's present state through stories, symbols, and metaphors to explore emotions and generate new perspectives. There is considerable crossover in the skills and techniques used in both functions. Shuttling between the two spheres with grace, the active intelligence of the nurse integrates the complementary function of both sides into a larger whole.

Essence: The Authentic Healing Presence of the Nurse

Systems of art and science are modified over time, creating and organizing new knowledge in terms of, and in response to, a specific set of issues or problems. The overarching evolutionary progress of humanity has always been towards higher order. In the past 300 years we have made vast strides in the worlds of art and science, learning to harness and distribute energy while creating new forms of machines, materials, and beauty. What has been slower in development is the subjective psycho/social/spiritual side of humanity. Our power to manipulate and control the outside world has advanced greatly, but we have not made similar advances in understanding our own behavior and our inner experience.

Current challenges facing society in general, and health care in particular, are pressing for a new way to comprehend and enhance the inner world of humankind. The lack of advances in understanding human behavior and inner experience have prevented us from solving pressing issues such as war, the world population explosion, and the poisoning of our planet. On a personal scale, we are experiencing the growth of lifestyle-related chronic illness at all ages and stages of the life continuum. Depression, mental illness, addiction, and obesity point to a culture deeply in search of meaning as old forms and processes fall away.

Conventional healing efforts have been focused into the past, trying to unearth the origins of patterns that do not serve us well. Health care professionals have traditionally helped people who are suffering to focus on contextual issues within their lives: family, career, social, and economic issues. However, the quantum perspective in healing offers us a new and transformative approach to illness and crisis. Stepping out of our life situation—becoming witness—opens up the present moment, the place where resolution resides.

When our mind is filled with problems, there is no room for anything new to enter, no room for a solution. Whenever we can create some space, we will find the life that exists underneath the situation, the life that is our birthright. In most people's normal state of awareness, they identify with their thought processes, reactions, desires, and aversions. Run by the ego, they are in a continuous low level of unease, discontent, boredom, or nervousness—a constant background static. This keeps them unaware and out of touch with the being side of their nature. They live in a state of inner pollution.

Becoming conscious occurs when we truly step into the moment. As we learn to witness our own thoughts and emotions, rather than being driven by them, we become surprised at the freedom in the world. Anything unconscious becomes conscious as we turn our focus towards it, and the light of our presence shines more brightly.

Nurses have long observed the spiritual dimension of healing, but little of this is captured in the medical record. Yet, we intuitively recognize that the spiritual side of human nature is an essential aspect of the healing process.

> There is a force that is unfathomable, omnipresent, unnamable and omniscient. This intelligent and loving force stands behind and guides the evolution of physical manifestation. Spirituality is the label used to describe what occurs when we connect with this source. (Unknown teacher)

The source of spirituality emerges from many names: Organizing Wisdom, Great Spirit, Creator, Christ Within, Atman, God, the Field, the Universal, the One. We connect to this source automatically, and often when least expected. Understanding spiritual truth occurs as we remove blocks to its recognition. Just as opening the blinds in a dark room allows the sunlight to pour in, opening to our innate spiritual nature invites the new and unexpected to emerge. In their compelling book, *The Spirituality of Imperfection,* Kurtz and Ketcham observed:

> Spirituality points, always, beyond: beyond the ordinary, beyond possession, beyond the narrow confines of self, and—above all—beyond expectation. Because the 'spiritual' is beyond control, it is never exactly what we expect. (Kurtz & Ketcham, 2002, p. 7)

Tapping into the deeper levels of being where our true innate intelligence resides requires bringing the spiritual dimension into the healing process. As we integrate our inner rhythms into our lives, we begin to experience a flowing interconnectedness around us that eventually includes the entire human and planetary family. Holistic physician Hogben notes:

> Healing may be defined as a miraculous unfolding of consciousness for one's being in the world. We learn who we are, what and who really matter

to us, how to express ourselves fully and openly. Ultimately the healing journey leads to an intimate union with the One through the experience of the flow of Spirit within. It is a slow, arduous passage, unique for each individual, filled with danger and risk, triumph and joy, and finally, peace, trust, awe, reverence, love and compassion. (Chopra, 1989, p. 94)

Healing goes beyond dealing with a health problem or crisis. It touches every aspect of life, facilitating a continuous movement towards wholeness and peace. In order to support the healing of others, we must also be on the path ourselves. Therefore, nurse and patient are partners in this expansive journey towards wholeness.

A health challenge creates an opening in time and space from which flow the inner feelings, hopes, intentions, expectations, memories, pain, and decisions that give depth and context to the person suffering. At this "edge of existence" lies the opportunity and the invitation to become more fully who we are.

Supporting the deeper soul work of healing, nurses assist people with physical and emotional challenges and fears in more authentic fashion. No longer do we analyze the event or look to the past or present circumstances for explanations. No longer do we foster resistance to weaknesses or deep feelings of sadness with will power or discipline. Instead, we help the person stay with their feelings and learn to observe them without reaction, description, or interpretation. In that open state, a relationship is created between the person and their true qualities or essence, opening up the possibility for real transformation and growth.

SELF-KNOWLEDGE: THE KEY TO HEALING PRESENCE

To offer a safe and open space for deep self-reflection, we must know our own self. This may involve the process of seeing where we came from just so we can let it go and move forward. A lovely paradox is found: while fear is always directed towards the future, that which haunts us—that which is creating the fear—is derived from the past.

This is not a call for perfection as that is an impossible goal. Once a student of Carl Rogers, noted psychologist and founder of the "person-centered approach to life," approached this noted therapist with a question: "How is it that every time I see you with a patient, any patient, they immediately open up to you with such candor?" Dr. Rogers replied, "Before I go into any room, I remind myself that I am not perfect. I am human. Therefore, I am capable of any thought/emotion/act that has ever been had. Being perfect is not enough. I am called to be human, and in that space I am one with all I meet" (Rogers, 1980, p. 121).

Socrates encouraged us to know ourselves. Knowing our own self in this deep sense includes the past as well as our true potential, which represents the future. As we move towards truly knowing our self and our inherent qualities, we are released from being haunted by the past that limits our freedom to be. Our true essence emerges, creating space for others to more fully touch their own.

Socrates was inviting us to have a relationship with ourselves, because then no one can haunt us or claim responsibility for who we are. True freedom comes through knowing our self, and *this does not require having to change anything.* All that is needed is to see what has been without reacting to it in any way. In so doing, we put an end to the story; we transcend our history to become the qualities, the real essence of our being. This is wholeness. And, once acquired in our life, we can hold space for others to find their own way home.

> *Give us grace, O God, to dare to do the deed which we well know cries to be done. Let us not hesitate because of ease, or the words of [people's] mouths, or our own lives. Mighty causes are calling us—the freeing of women, the training of children, the putting down of hate and murder and poverty—all these and more. But they call with voices that mean work and sacrifice and death. May we find a way to meet the task.*
>
> W.E.B. Du Bois

BIBLIOGRAPHY

Bohm, D., & Hiley, B. (1993). *The undivided universe: An ontological interpretation of quantum theory.* New York: Routledge.

Briskin, A. (2005). *Rishi.* Oakland, CA: Unpublished manuscript.

Calabria, M. D., & Macrae, J. A. (1994). *Suggestions for thought by Florence Nightingale: Selections and commentaries.* Philadelphia: University of Philadelphia Press.

Capra, F. (1996). *The web of life: A new scientific understanding of living systems.* New York: Doubleday Dell.

Chopra, D. (1989). *Quantum healing.* New York: Bantam.

Gleck, J. (1987). *Chaos: Making a new science.* New York: Penguin.

Heisenberg, W. (1971). *Physics and beyond.* New York: Harper and Row.

Kurtz, E., & Ketcham, K. (2002). *The spirituality of imperfection: Storytelling and the search for meaning.* New York: Bantam.

Marshall, S. (2005, September–November). A decidedly different mind. *Shift: At the frontiers of consciousness,* (8), 14–17.

McTaggart, L. (2002). *The field.* New York: HarperCollins.

Nadeau, R., & Kafatos, M. (2002). *The non-local universe: The new physics and matter of the mind.* New York: Oxford University Press.

Pribram, K. H. (1991). *Brain and perception: Holomony and structure in figural processing.* Hillsdale, NJ: Lawrence Erlbaum.

Rogers, C. (1980). *A way of being.* Boston: Houghton Mifflin.

Shlain, L. (1991). *Art and physics: Parallel visions in space, time and light.* New York: Simon and Schuster.

Sussman, L. (1995). *Speech of the grail.* New York: Lindisfarne Press.

Suzuki, D. (2002). *The sacred balance: Rediscovering our place in nature.* Vancouver, CA: Graystone Books.

Vaill, P. (1996). *Learning as a way of being.* San Francisco: Jossey-Bass.

SECTION II

A Healing Field: The Context for Nursing Practice

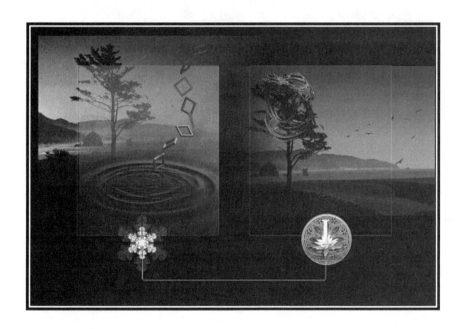

Happiness is being at peace with your self
while the self is united with a larger
order of things, for we live in the world
which is a sanctuary.

Henryk Skolimowski

CHAPTER 2

The Noetic Scientist

A Holistic Worldview

Scientists do not invent the truth, they discover it.
Genuine truths exude a beauty,
a rightness, a self-evident quality
that gives them the power of revelation.

John Horgan

We are living in the twilight of the scientific age. Conventional science is a science of objects; its theories regard objects in terms of other, more fundamental, objects, with controlled predictability of behavior and outcomes. While the scientific community differs on their answers to the question: what is life beyond biological functioning? scientific advances pose increasing limitations upon science itself. Ironically, as scientific discovery progresses it is beginning to realize the ultimate *limits of knowledge;* it may be ending because it has worked so well (Hogan, 1996).

Increasingly, scientists from various disciplines cast their gaze across the field, and find that for all its power and richness, it cannot explain the ultimate mystery of consciousness; the link between mind and matter. The enlarging voice of quantum physicists postulates that the key to this deep divide lies in the fissure between two major theories of modern physics: quantum mechanics—which describes nuclear forces and electromagnetism, and general relativity—Einstein's theory of gravity (Penrose, 1994).

EXPANDING OUR SCIENCE: HOLISM VERSUS REDUCTIONISM

For the past 400 years, Western civilization has looked to science as its source of truths and wisdom regarding the mysteries of life. In 1543, Copernicus's observations regarding reality began a scientific revolution that was later defined by Newton. The Newtonian classical physics-based deterministic worldview fostered a materialistic mind-set that saw the world as an intricate mechanism with separate parts and processes. The scientist's job was to discover the thread that unifies and weaves the separate entities into a unified whole through a process of *reductionism*—taking matter apart and studying its bits and pieces. In this model *causation flows upward,* from the base level of elementary particles (Goswami, 2004).

Elementary particles create atoms, which in turn form molecules, which configure together to produce a cell. Cells generate all of the energies of the body. Some of the cells create neurons, which in turn construct the brain. The brain generates mental processes in the upper levels of physiological hierarchy. Knowledge of the universe's parts and their interaction allows scientists to predict and control nature. Control is the principle function of *determinism,* the belief that with knowledge of something's parts we can predict its behavior. This materialistic and deterministic worldview fosters a dualistic perspective, a split between mind and matter, which can be controlled and managed through the laws of science. It supports the idea that humans are disconnected from, and are above, nature.

This reductionistic approach to understanding the nature of the universe has bestowed valuable knowledge, which created the space age, artificial hearts and limbs, and deciphering of the genetic code. However, applying those same principles to business, health care, and world problems is hastening a local and global crisis. Therefore, leading-edge scientific research is beginning to question fundamental assumptions long held as dogma by conventional science.

The discovery of the quantum world put an end to certainty. Prigogine and other scientists noted that chaos and complexity offer a different vision of the world than the mechanistic view of traditional science. This world is filled with fluidity, multiplicity, plurality, connectedness, segmentarity, heterogeneity, and resilience. *Downward causation, mind over matter,* originates from the intentions and thoughts of the individual, rather than some outside force. The notion of scientific knowledge is replaced with the concept of *self-organizing dynamics* of nonorganic, organic, and social phenomena. Determinism is replaced with *emergence* of new order as this chaotic phenomenon is supported, rather than controlled, by links between order and disorder as new form materializes (Prigogine & Stengers, 1984). The underlying assumption is that to understand nature and the human experience we must transcend the parts to see the interconnected whole.

The impact of a radically new worldview challenges the very foundations of medical and nursing practice. Western medicine traditionally conceptualized the body as a grand machine, controlled by the brain and peripheral nervous system: the ultimate biological computer. Human physiology and psychological behavior were viewed as dependent upon the structure and hardware of brain and body, with a mechanical heart pump to deliver nutrients to all body cells.

This traditional viewpoint has been expanding since Einstein's discovery introduced the concept that all matter is an expression of energy. Einstein stepped beyond reductionism towards holism, showing that both matter and energy are expressions of the same universal substance (Einstein, 1952). The recognition that all matter is energy, $E = mc^2$, forms the foundation for understanding how human beings can be considered dynamic energetic systems. In this world, human beings are viewed as networks of complex energy fields that interface with physical/cellular systems (McTaggart, 2002). Therefore, healing of this basic vibrational energetic level of substance can be accomplished through multiple therapeutic venues beyond traditional medicine.

In spite of a growing field of evidence, present-day Newtonian models of medical thinking still prevail in the practice of conventional medicine, the context for contemporary nursing practice. We are being called to re-envision our world and our work by embracing the best of tradition while expanding our worldview to encompass the larger quantum world of holism.

ENLARGING OUR PRACTICE:
EXPANSIVE SCIENTIFIC MODELS

Lipton (2005–2006) notes that over the centuries scientists have constructed their knowledge into a hierarchical, multitiered building. Each level, distinguished by a specific sub-specialty, is built upon the supporting structures of lower levels. We are now invited to "enlarge our living room" by incorporating the tools and processes of the quantum world into our world and our work.

The foundation for integrative science is laid on the first floor of fractals and chaos. Mathematical laws have traditionally been used to isolate and divide the universe into separate measurable components. Future science will also include the emerging new math, which emphasizes the disciplines of fractal geometry, chaos theory, and fuzzy logic (Kosko, 1993). Bohm also suggests that the new research tool is dialogue rather than statistics. In true dialogue multiple perspectives are shared and something organic, emerging and new, is discovered in the shared space (Bohm & Peat, 1987).

Fractals, the modern version of geometry, were defined by IBM scientist Benoit Mandelbrot (1977). This simple mathematic equation involves addition and multiplication, with the results being entered back into the original equation and solved again. Repetition of the equation provides for a geometric expression of self-similar objects that appear at higher or lower levels of magnitude. Like nested Russian dolls, organization at any level of nature reflects a self-similar pattern at higher and lower levels of reality. The structure and function of a cell reflects behavior of a human, group, and society. "As above, so below" is emphasized, showing that the observable physical universe is derived from the interconnectivity and integration of all its parts.

Displacing the Darwinian evolution theory based on mutations and a struggle for survival, fractal geometry demonstrates that the biosphere is a very structured and cooperative venture among all living organisms. Rather than competition for survival, nature models cooperation among species living in harmony with their environment. It highlights the fact that every being counts; we are all members of a single organism.

The dynamics of fractal structures, from mountains to clouds to plants to humans, are directly influenced by chaos theory (Gleick, 1988). This math transcends predictability and control, showing that a small change may cause unexpected final outcomes. Combining chaos theory with fractal geometry, the behavioral dynamics in physical reality can only be predicted within a reference range of possible outcomes rather than controlled.

The second floor of science explores energy physics. A century ago a group of creative minorities in the field of quantum mechanics transcended the Newtonian view of the universe as an assembly of physical parts. Albert Einstein, Max Planck, and Werner Heisenberg, among others, revealed that there is no true physicality in the universe (Hawking, 1988). Atoms are miniature tornados of energy, popping in and out of existence. They create energy fields that encompass the universe, closely entangled with each other and the field that contains them all.

A radical conclusion of the new physics recognizes that the observer creates the reality. Through the power of observation, each of us personally creates our own reality! This knowing forces physicists to acknowledge that the universe is a mental construct. Physicist Sir James Jean observed that "The stream of knowledge is heading toward a nonmechanical reality; the universe begins to look more like a great thought than like a great machine" (Henry, 2005). While this knowledge was uncovered 80 years ago, many scientists cling rigidly to the prevailing matter-oriented worldview. We are being called to recognize that our beliefs, perceptions, and attitudes about the world create that world for us.

The third floor of science focuses on vibrational chemistry. Conventional chemistry was built on atomic elements of solid electrons, protons, and neutrons within a Newtonian solar system. Vibrational chemistry is derived from quantum mechanics, which view atoms as spinning, immaterial energy vortices called quarks. It sees vibration as the process that creates molecular bonds and drives molecular interactions. Energy fields, such as those emerging from outside sources like cell phones, or the interior world of thoughts and emotions, interact with and influence chemical reactions (Tsong, 1989).

Mind-body connection is mediated by the mechanisms fostered by vibrational chemistry. The body is created from a hundred thousand different protein molecules, which change shape in response to signals. These harmonic vibrations in the field influence the collective movement of the protein body, generating the behaviors we observe as life.

Life-controlling signals originate from physical chemicals as well as energy waves. This energy-protein interface is the junction of the mind-body connection (Pert, 1997).

The fourth floor of science focuses on the new biology. In traditional biology, in reductionistic fashion, organisms are dissected into cells and molecular parts to gain understanding of how they work. The new science perceives cells as integrated communities that are physically and energetically entangled within their environment (Gerber, 1996). James Lovelock's hypothesis states that our Earth and its biosphere comprise a single living and breathing entity, which he calls Gaia. Gaian philosophy emphasizes participation and integration of all the earth's organisms to maintain homeostasis and balance (Lovelock, 1979).

A second new field of biology is the power of epigenetics. This field, which means "control above the genes," addresses the newly uncovered second genetic code, which controls the activity and programming of DNA. A heredity mechanism, it reveals how behavior and gene activity are controlled by the organism's perception of its environment. Moving from the determinism of DNA coding, epigenetics recognizes the role of our perceptions, including emotions and consciousness, in controlling our genes. Applied consciousness can be used to shape our biology, making us masters of our own lives (Lipton, 2005).

The fifth floor of science focuses on energy psychology. For centuries our materialistic perspective has dismissed the immaterial mind and consciousness, perceiving instead that our genes and neurochemicals—the hardware of our central nervous system, were responsible for behavior and dysfunction alike. Quantum mechanics, vibrational chemistry, and epigenetics offer a new understanding of psychology.

The environment, coupled with perceptions of the mind and their resultant emotions and feelings, controls behavior and genetics. Our lives are controlled by our perceptions of life experiences rather than by genetic programming (Mindel, 2004). Moving from Newtonian to quantum mechanics shifts the focus of psychology from physiochemical mechanisms to energy fields. This altered understanding moves us away from psychological interventions targeted at physiochemical hardware, genetic manipulation, altered physiology, and behavior modification. An enlarged focus on energy psychology recognizes the power of fundamental perceptions, leading to the creation of deepening developmental experiences as a therapeutic intervention. A new perspective can enhance our health, intelligence, and happiness, shifting our values and moral code to a higher order. Focusing on our potential and our capacity moves us forward into a fuller life, rather than backwards to a limiting history.

By remodeling each "floor" of our house of science, we strengthen the building while adding an observatory on the top. From this vantage point our worldview is holistic; the view of a *noetic scientist*. The word *noetic,* coming from ancient Greece, refers to an inner knowing, an intuitive consciousness that is direct and immediate, allowing us access to knowledge beyond what is available to our normal senses and our patterns of reasoning (www.noetic.org). Here we *know* that the physical character of atoms, proteins, cells, and people are all influenced by immaterial energies that form a collective field. Each human, a collective cellular community, responds to a unique spectrum of the universe's energy field. This unique spectrum, referred to by many as Spirit, signifies an invisible moving force that is in harmonic resonance with our physical body. This profound, creative force behind consciousness shapes our physical reality.

We also note that collectively we are a part of a larger, shared field that cocreates our reality. As this understanding deepens, our relationship with the planet becomes one of partnership. We begin to live lightly on the earth, using only the resources we need while practicing principles that support sustainability. We live responsibly, moving with care and compassion through the world.

RECREATING OUR REALITY:
NURSES AS NOETIC SCIENTISTS

To resolve local and global crisis requires us to re-envision conventional science through the integration and coordination of both the physical/material world and the energetic/immaterial world. Healing and wholeness will come through the support and services of *cultural creatives,* a minority of healers who practice from an integrative view of themselves and the world.

We live in a time of great promise as we have developed economic and social systems that tap human creativity as never before. The great dilemma of our time is the fact that we lack the broader social and economic systems to fully harness it and put it to use.

The number of people doing creative work that will transform society has been steadily increasing, especially in the past two decades. These pioneers of the new age, working as scientists, engineers, artists, and knowledge-based professionals such as nurses, are referred to as the "Creative Class" (Florida, 2002, p. 3).

Creative nurses have always been in our midst, living an experiential lifestyle. Our history is rich with their presence, starting with Florence Nightingale. The foundation for nursing's work is science first and foremost; applied science is our practice domain. The mind-set of a contemporary scientist is reflected in the clinical reasoning capacity of this nurse. The nurse is focused on finding answers that get somewhere; the nurse cannot tolerate untestable speculation. The creative is eager to share his or her knowledge in an effort to make things as clear as possible, and to expand her or his understanding through networking with similar colleagues. Free of self-doubt, wishful thinking, and deep attachment to specific theories or protocols, this applied scientist simply comes from a stance of wanting to know how things work to create a positive affect for the patient.

A study by Rich Florida (2002) demonstrated that in 1900 less than 1% of American workers were doing creative work. By 1980 the figure was still well below 10%. Today, more than 30% of the nation's workforce is shaping the profound shifts in the ways we work, in our values and desires, and the very fabric of our lives. Capacities of those who live on the edge as agents of change inside traditional professional jobs include:

- Technology—these nurses embrace, seek out, and create solutions that utilize emerging technologies (new tools and resources, both material and ideological) to extend their capacity.
- Talent—these nurses not only demonstrate clinical and technical skill and aptitude, but a creative and adventuresome capacity for innovation and experimentation.
- Tolerance—these nurses have an edge in the ability to attract different kinds of people who generate new ideas and methods for responding to the work before them.

Cultural creatives engage an active imagination. Quantum scientist Minsky confessed he would love to know what Yo-Yo Ma felt as he was playing a concert, doubting whether such an experience were possible. To do so he would have to have all of Yo-Yo Ma's memories; he would have to *become* Yo-Yo Ma. But in becoming Yo-Yo Ma, he would cease to be Minsky. No such reduction is possible because multiplicity of the mind is the human birthright.

The cultural creatives who have mastered many skills during their careers have learned to enjoy the feeling of awkwardness triggered by having to learn something new. There is no sense of failure when things do not work out, rather the delight of experimentation and discovery that is present in children. Minsky further stated, "It's so thrilling not to be able to do something. It's such a rare experience to treasure, and it won't last long" (Hogan, 1996, pp. 188–189). He observed that the most important thing in life is to grow beyond our current state, to become more our essential self. This is the grand opportunity called life.

Resourceful nurses thrive in a broad ecosystem that nourishes and supports creativity and channels it into innovation that eventually changes practice within the discipline.

Such nurses have always worked on the margins, expanding the field on behalf of the people we are privileged to serve. The key to their survival is to squelch the squelchers: the controlling leaders, micromanagers, and broader structures of social control and vertical power. The real threat to America is not terrorism, but rather the suppression of the creative and talented people who have a commitment and capacity to enrich the world in which we live.

The power of this cultural scientific revolution lies in a nurse's ability to select the "best-of-breed" ideas and innovations and blend them in novel ways. People with differing perspectives contribute their own original ideas into the boiling stew, creating new thought. Connection and collaboration are the tools of the information age that are essential for the creatives in our midst.

For thousands of years human evolution was limited to the very slow pace of genetic evolution. Cultural scientific evolution is much faster, because what is learned can be passed on through language. Beginning with the development of the alphabet and then the printing press, the emergence of the Internet has put wings on communication in ways that transcend time and distance.

Just as cultural evolution learned to operate independently of biological evolution, so too is Web-based evolution becoming autonomous. The intellectual impact of this interconnected world is fostering a renaissance greater than any shift in the history of humankind. Even scientists and specialists are increasingly taking the word of electronic circuits for critical information on vital issues.

By processing information adaptively, the nurse of the twenty-first century will open up important new vistas for health and healing to the people she or he serves. Patients and families will absorb the new and enlarging information through their experiences around health, adjusting themselves accordingly. Their tomorrows will turn out different from their todays, for increased understanding leaves us free to evolve in whatever fashion works best for each of us. And in the process of shared growth and understanding, the world will become a healing place.

> *I will not die an unlived life.*
> *I will not live in fear*
> *Of falling or catching fire.*
> *I choose to inhabit my days,*
> *To allow my living to open me,*
> *To make me less afraid,*
> *More accessible,*

To loosen my heart
Until it becomes a wing,
A torch, a promise.
I choose to risk my significance;
To live so that which came to me as seed
Goes to the next as blossom
And that which came to me as blossom,
Goes on as fruit.

Dawna Markova

BIBLIOGRAPHY

Bohm, D., & Peat, E. F. (1987). *Science, order and creativity.* New York: Bantam.

Einstein, A. (1952). *The principle of relativity: A collection of original papers on the special and general theory of relativity.* New York: Dover.

Florida, R. (2002). *The rise of the creative class: And how it's transforming work, leisure, community and everyday life.* New York: Basic Books.

Gerber, R. (1996). *Vibrational medicine.* Santa Fe, NM: Bear and Company.

Gleick, J. (1988). *Chaos: Making a new science.* New York: Penguin.

Goswami, A. (2004). *The quantum doctor: A physicist's guide to health and healing.* Charlottesville, VA: Hampton Roads.

Hawking, S. (1988). *A brief history of time: From the big bang to black holes.* London: Bantam.

Henry, R. C. (2005). The mental universe. *Nature, 436,* 29, p. 71.

Hogan, J. (1996). *The end of science.* New York: Broadway Books.

Kosko, B. (1993). *Fuzzy thinking: The new science of fuzzy logic.* New York: Hyperion.

Lipton, B. (2005). *The biology of belief: Unleashing the power of consciousness, matter and miracles.* Santa Rosa, CA: Mountain of Love/Elite Books.

Lipton, B. (2005–2006, December–February). Embracing the immaterial universe. *Shift: At the Frontiers of Consciousness,* (9), 8–12.

Lovelock, J. (1979). *Gaia: A new look at life on Earth.* Oxford: Oxford University Press.

Mandelbrot, B. (1977). *The fractal geometry of nature.* San Francisco: W. H. Freeman.

McTaggart, L. (2002). *The field.* New York: HarperCollins.

Mindel, A. (2004). *The quantum mind and healing.* Charlottesville, VA: Hampton Roads.

Penrose, R. (1994). *Shadows of the mind.* New York: Oxford University Press.

Pert, C. (1997). *Molecules of emotion: Why you feel the way you feel.* New York: Scribner.

Prigogine, I., & Stengers, I. (1984). *Order out of chaos.* New York: Bantam.

Tsong, T. Y. (1989). Deciphering the language of cells. *Trends in Biochemical Sciences* 149 (14), 89.

CHAPTER 3

The Creative Artist

Composing a Life

Einstein's space is no closer to reality than Van Gogh's sky. The glory of science is not in a truth more absolute than the truth of Bach or Tolstoy, but in the act of creation itself. The scientist's discoveries impose his own order on chaos, as the composer or painter imposes his; an order that always refers to limited aspects of reality, and is based on the observer's frame of reference, which differs from period to period as a Rembrandt nude differs from a nude by Manet.

Arthur Koestler

Each of us is born into a culture whose orientations and basic beliefs shape us, and they remain deeply rooted in our personality for all of our life. As we move beyond home and hearth we find differing cultures and beliefs that we can incorporate into our understanding of the world. However, those first roots remain deep and immovable, no matter how we try to shake or transcend them.

This same phenomenon is observed within a field of knowledge. The sources that gave birth to the field remain within it as a skeleton that organizes the shape of things, defining in part what is real and true, what embodies the basic essence of reality from that point of view.

When we, or a field, encounter new data that contradicts our old beliefs and basic orientation, a struggle of confusion arises. There is increasing difficulty in communication between those within the family or the field. Early adaptors will incorporate some of the new into their world and work, while a small segment will die without ever acknowledging that anything could ever change. For the majority, however, there is a dance between old and new, past and future, with a slow drift towards the pole that attracts us most.

The reality that comprises our world of observation can be divided into differing realms of experience, each with a different level of awareness.

1. *Consensus reality* is comprised of observations of time, space, weight, and repeatable measures and behaviors. Cause-and-effect activities of things that can be seen or touched comprise this domain, which is validated by the science and culture of the times. We engage with this world as the evaluator.

2. *Inner reality* is comprised of highly individualized inner experiences of fantasies, subjective feelings, emotions, and dreams. We create meaning from the projections and interpretations that we selectively or habitually weave into our experiences coming from the outer world. Captured through the contributions of the arts, we experience this world as the interpreter.

3. *Core essence* is a perception of the subtle energy field behind the form being observed. In this space is a clear sense of the force of silence from which all things arise, including an awareness of things too big to be touched (macrocosm), as well as those too small to be seen (microcosm), even theoretically. This field is the universal sacred space of Spirit addressed by philosophy and religion. To perceive this world requires us to become the witness to things invisible that cannot be named.

Science explores the reality of the physical world, while art focuses on experiences of inner reality. Philosophy and religion give shape and direction to the realm of essence, influencing the moral ethics of the times (Leshan & Margenau, 1982). Together, these things form and inform, bringing beauty and meaning to the human journey. Each of these realms is experienced uniquely as an individual, and collectively as the human family. But the continuing explorations and discoveries in art, science, and philosophy keep redefining these domains, inviting us to continue expanding our own capacities for understanding, creating an expansion of consciousness.

Art and physics fashion a strange partnership, yet they are the forces that define and unite our objective and subjective worlds together. The artist creates a world of image and metaphor, while the physicist employs numbers and equations. Art embraces the imaginative reality of aesthetic qualities, while physics shuttles between a world of specific mathematical relationships and quantifiable properties. Art creates illusions to elicit emotion, while physics strives to create an exact and predictable science. However, when closely examined, both are an effort at investigating the nature of reality to create a fuller understanding of life. Noted physicist David Bohm observed that "Physics is a form of insight and as such it's a form of art" (Shlain, 1991, p. 78).

While the scientific side of the nursing practice breaks things into component parts to establish a relationship between them, the artisan juxtaposes different distinct and unique features of the particular patient and his or her circumstance, synthesizing them into a larger whole. There is considerable crossover in this sacred work of weaving the scientific with the psychospiritual.

ART: THE POWER OF PERSPECTIVE

Radical innovations in art embody the preverbal stages of new concepts that hold potential to change the outcome of an external event, group, or society. A new way to think about reality begins with the assimilation of unfamiliar images that leads to abstract ideas that later give rise to specific words and/or actions. When we reflect, reminisce, ruminate, and imagine, we are generally in the visual mode. However, in order to perform the brain's highest function, abstract thought, we must move to the realm of essence—energy before form. Here we go beyond the use of images, engaging our intuition and intent to create in a world that transcends image and language.

Notably, it is images that precede abstract thought and descriptive language. Artist Paul Klee observed that "The artist does not reproduce the visible; rather he makes things visible" (Chipp, 1956, p. 182). Picasso said, "I see for others" (Reed, 1968, p. 87). Nurses are both artist in their trade, and observer in the gallery of another's masterpiece—their life. When they enter the nurse-patient experience with respect for the person, the nurse recognizes that, as life artist, the person has crafted their life in the way that seems best to them. Without judgment, the compassionate professional stands alongside the person and family as they view the situation at hand, incorporating new information and issues into the landscape of their existence. Goeth observed:

> Works of art specify no immediate action or limited use. They are like gateways, where the visitor [nurse as interpreter] can enter the space of the artist [patient-family], or the time of the poet [context-culture], to experience whatever rich domain [life] the artist has fashioned. (Quoted in Dowson, 1979, p. 26)

Art and physics, like wave and particle, weave together to form an articulation of the clinical reasoning process that gives the interpreter function of nursing a profound place of importance in the healing experience. This recognition of an understated phenomenon and an immediate proactive response can alter the ultimate outcome and future-state for all involved (Pesut & Herman, 1999).

Multidimensionality: The Influence of Time and Space

One of the great gifts of art is the opportunity to see the world through perspectives other than our own. Many artistic styles have evolved throughout history, depicting our deepening perception of time and space, and humankind's place within it.

A *zero-dimensional world* is expressed in the simplest geometric object; a point. Without size, it can only be imagined. It fixes a location in space with a dimension that equals zero.

When this point gets extended into a simple line, it has only *one dimension*—length. The first recorded art forms were created on the walls of cave dwellings in the form of stick figures and objects. One-dimensional beings perceive the world as points only, with no sense of a self who resides outside the points.

A *two-dimensional world* includes the concept of a plane—a surface. In this universe things have breadth and width, while still lacking height. Two-dimensional beings can encounter lines, or barriers, with time experienced as the moment. Since this space is a flatland, any barrier must be walked around, for there is no space to jump or step over the object. Byzantine art in the late fifth and early sixth centuries depicted individuals and figures on a flat background. Depth and movement were attempted by depicting the same figure in multiple poses surrounding the central figure, or by breaking them down into small pieces of mosaic.

Three-dimensional space includes matter—a solid body that adds the perspective of height or mass, and linear time marching progressively forward. The generation of Renaissance painters perfected the creation of a broad view from a single perspective by incorporating the third dimension in depth painting. In these art forms an object painted on a flat surface was given the perception of depth by making objects appear to have the same size, shape, and position in relation to each other. In such a picture the road diminishes in size and prominence as it moves back into the horizon, while smaller trees dot the background with the larger in the foreground. Great masters, including such notables as Da Vinci and Michelangelo, left many images of beauty for us in this three-dimensional realm of length, breadth, and depth (Shlain, 1991, p. 24). See Figure 3.1.

A three-dimensional being can see only two dimensions, while humans can note all three. Because we can delineate external forms in three dimensions and manipulate three-dimensional spaces, we must recognize the truth; that *we are four-dimensional beings* (Steiner, 2001, pp. 8–10, 40–42).

By adding the fourth dimension of multiple possibilities, everyday three-dimensional space is transformed into a four-dimensional hyperspace that is

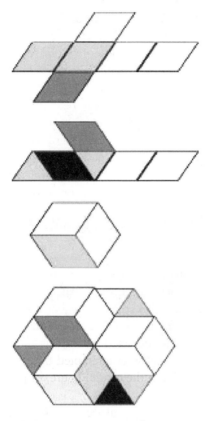

FIGURE 3.1   Dimensions of space-time.

infused with an unlimited vista including the past, the future, and the time-less. In this extending view, you become aware of your observer self witness-ing a larger reality. You begin to note an ongoing process moving between and through yourself as well as all other states of being.

Early artists of this movement included masters such as Monet, who painted 40 different pictures of one chapel door to show changes in time of day and seasons of the year. However, each picture remained a single portrait of a stationary object with the viewer standing outside, looking in.

A recent Norman Rockwell art exhibit featured some of his most famous works. Instead of the traditional art show of original paintings, this exhibit also offered several life-size models built to allow the viewer to enter the pic-ture, interact with it, and experience it from multiple perspectives.

The story captured in the picture *Surprise,* which appeared on the *Saturday Evening Post* cover in March, 1956, occurs in a one-room schoolhouse. You enter the school through the back door, stepping behind several rows of desks to the backs of the children facing a blackboard. Miss Jones is standing in front of the room, gazing at the children with delight and affection mirrored in her eyes. The blackboard holds multiple messages of "Surprise," "Happy Birthday Miss Jones," "Miss Jones is our favorite teacher," and so on.

Walking down the aisle, you may stop and sit in a student desk. When the desk lid is lifted, one sees a small slate blackboard, chalk, books, and a wide-awake toad that was captured at recess. Arriving at the front of the room, you may take your place beside Miss Jones and see the excitement and joy on the faces of the children. Opening her desk you find a collection of teaching materials, along with an abundance of slingshots and paper wads with rubber bands. You may write on the board, adding your own greeting to this beloved teacher.

After you have walked through and experienced the perspective of each of the major characters in the picture, you have a deep and rich sense of what it must have been like to be both the student and teacher in an era of greater simplicity. You may recall similar moments in your own childhood, whether at school or with parents or grandparents, when you crafted a surprise to show appreciation for someone's guiding presence in your life. An artifact in a desk or on the wall can trigger emotions and thoughts that have not been examined for many years. You may recall your own school experiences, or ponder how vastly different the education of your grandchildren will be with the advent of the Internet and the ease of global travel.

As you walk through the painting, you select items of interest. You and each object you relate to are intimate, connected in a pure and nondualistic way. You become both yourself and the object towards which you move. In the end, you have reflected on something larger than yourself, a phenomenon that spans both time and distance. Deeper understanding and meaning are possible from this point of view (Russell, 1974, p. 31).

In fourth-dimensional space, half of the experience—objects and the light that illumines them—are objectively given. The other two dimensions—emotions and interpretation—are subjectively experienced. The further we move into other dimensions, the more subjective the experience becomes. What lies within the higher worlds can only be attained through the development of new envisioning possibilities. We must become active in accessing and understanding these worlds, rather than being passive viewers only.

Physicists are now exploring "hyperspace," and have identified as many as 10 differing dimensions, including wormholes, superstrings, and parallel universes (Kaku, 1994). While mathematicians, physicists, and computers have no problem solving theoretical problems in multidimensional space, humans find it impossible to visualize universes beyond their own four-dimensional world.

Artist photographers are giving us new images of the macrocosm with pictures from the Hubble spacecraft that are startling in their beauty and magnitude. Contemporary filmmakers working with computer-assisted graphics are creating compelling epic movies such as *Lord of the Rings* and *Harry Potter,* endowing humans with superhuman capacities. Popular motion pictures also create awareness of things unseen through stories, such as *The Matrix, Brother Bear,* and *Atlantis.* Action-oriented art forms such as these are heralding a new way of being in multiple worlds simultaneously, opening up and modeling new possibilities and capacities for the next generation of humanity.

One fundamental theme running through the findings in physics over the past decade is this: "The laws of nature become simpler and more elegant when expressed in higher dimensions, which is their natural home" (Kaku, 1994, p. 12). In higher order, as the number of dimensions in space-time increase, more forces can be accommodated. Here we have enough room to unify all of the known physical forces: electromagnetic, strong nuclear, weak nuclear, and gravitational forces. When these laws, which seem to have no relationship in three-dimensional space, are viewed in their natural habitat in the dimensions beyond space and time, their true brilliance and power can be observed and appreciated. The laws become simple and powerful—and beautiful.

The revolution sweeping over physics is the realization that we do not have the technology or the money to prove (in the traditional sense) the reality of these far-reaching dimensions. Because it is untestable, scientists are asking this question: "*Is beauty, by itself, a physical principle that can be substituted for the lack of experimental verification?*" (Kaku, 1994, p. 179). Suddenly, the physicist is an artist! Nobel Prize winner Sheldon Glashow of Harvard penned this poem:

> The Theory of Everything, if you dare to be bold,
> Might be something more than a string orbitfold.
> While some of your leaders have got old and sclerotic,
> Not to be trusted alone with things heterotic,
> Please heed our advice that you are not smitten—
> The Book is not finished, the last word is not Written.
> (Glashow, 1988, p. 335)

Science is young, only 400 years old, while art is ancient, preceding the emergence of language among the human species. And both are moving back/forward to a natural connection with the nature of life. Abram has observed that, "without the oxygenating breath of the forests, the clutch of gravity, we have no distance from our technologies, no way of assessing their limitations, no way of keeping ourselves from turning into them . . . only when we are in regular contact with the tangible ground and sky can we learn how to orient and to navigate in the multiple dimensions that now claim us" (Abram, 1996, p. x). This is the gift of the artist; artists give life and articulation to the essence of things of nature and spirit.

PATTERN: THE POWER OF LIMITS

The nurse artist has an exceptional capacity to recognize pattern and rhythm, as well as typical modifications induced by illness. She or he has taken an innate gift possessed by all at birth and enhanced a capacity for its application in professional practice.

Apple blossoms always have five petals and hands host five digits. When we look deeply into the patterns of a blossom, a seashell, or a song we discover a perfection of order that reveals an infinity greater than our own. Between the borders of art, science, religion, and philosophy lies a power that shapes our universe, our lives and our values: the golden mean. "The proportions in art, nature and the human body are shared limitations that create harmonious relationships out of differences. Limitations are not just restrictive, they are also creative" (Doczi, 1994, p. 27). See Figure 3.2.

There is discipline inherent in the patterns of natural phenomena, manifest in the most ageless and harmonious works of humanity in art, music, architecture, and social systems. Order emerges as certain proportions appear again and again, showing a dynamic growth pattern through a union of complementary opposites. Old and new stages of growth always share the same angles and proportions. The formula of the celebrated *golden mean:* A:B = B:(A+B), implies a reciprocal relationship between two unequal parts of a whole, wherein the smaller part stands in the same proportion to the larger part as the larger part stands to the whole (Doczi, 1994, p. 2).

Patterns typically generate spirals that move in opposite directions, forming a union of complementary opposites—sun and moon, yin and yang, male and female, positive and negative energy. This pattern-forming process creates an energy, a generative power called *dinergy: the creative energy of organic growth.* This energy-creating process transforms discrepancies into harmonies by allowing differences to complement each other through the power of certain proportions, analogous to musical root harmonies. Its power lies in the unique capacity to unite the differing parts into a whole that preserves the identity of each while blending them into a greater pattern of a single larger whole—an infinite number of times. Herein lies the foundation of cosmic

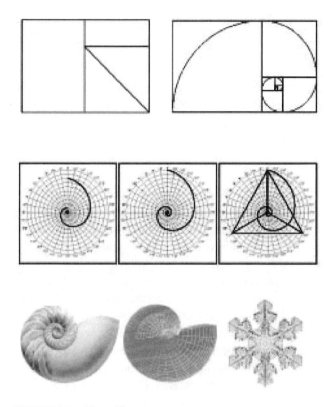

FIGURE 3.2   The golden mean.

order expressed in numerous mathematical equations and spiritual geometry (Doczi, 1994, p. 13).

Reality unites and diversifies at the same time. Poetry, painting, and the arts are given as a way for us to uncover the unity present in the variety of our human experiences. While there is no event or shape exactly the same, there is none entirely different from another. Nature accomplishes the most impossible feat: simultaneously creating forms that are both similar and dissimilar, united and diverse. This is what helps us distinguish human from animal and person from person; all are variations of the golden mean's proportions. Its simple aesthetic contribution is based on its direct relation to order and its inverse relation to complexity (Doczi, 1994, p. 25).

The ratio of dinergy is present in the crafts, the masterfully woven ceremonial blankets of First Nations artists, the delicate painting on a Chinese vase, the proportions of the human body in the sculpture of David. It is heard in musical creations based on a seven-tone scale, combined in endless iterations for song and dance, and in the written word based on shared meaning. The number seven is the primary harmonic quality. There are seven colors in the spectrum of a prism, seven notes in the musical scale, seven days in the week, seven chakras in the human body. The Lakota Sioux speak of the seven sacred directions: north, south, east, west, above, below, and the seventh sacred direction of the heart directly connected to Creator.

The ratio of dinergy is present in mathematical calculations from the Fibonacci numbers series to the architectural wonders of the world built from carefully calculated drawings. It is present everywhere in nature, from the pattern in a flower to the design of our DNA. Unity within the diversities of organic and inorganic matter can be seen in the spiral patterns of the galaxies, the tiny spiral pattern found in shells, flowers, and pine cones and the spiral pattern on our fingertips.

The science of nursing is focused on the functioning of the physical body, which is assessed and managed by diagnostic measurements and protocol-driven treatments. The art of nursing is concerned with the subtle aspects of care, noting a shift in pattern, a change in affect, an unstated concern expressed in body movements and facial expression displayed on both the foreground and background of the human landscape.

Leonardo Da Vinci created his famous drawing (see Figure 3.3) when the Renaissance rediscovered the classic remains of Greece and Rome:

> For if a man be placed flat on his back, with his hands and feet extended, and a pair of compasses entered at his navel, the fingers and toes of his two hands and feet will touch the circumference of a circle described therefrom. And just as the human body yields a circular outline, so, too, a square figure may be found from it. For if we measure the distance from the soles of the feet to the top of the head, and then apply that measure to the outstretched arms, the breadth will be found to be the same as the height, as in the case of plane surfaces which are perfectly square.... The circumference of the circle is approximately equal to the periphery of the square. (Vetruvius, quoted in Fischer, 1996a, p. 26)

"Squaring the circle," an archetypal idea from the mystery schools of Egypt, was based on shapes considered perfect and sacred. The circle represents a symbol of heavenly orbits, while the square depicts the foursquare firmness of the earth. Placing a body image into the center of the superimposed shapes depicts a metaphor for unity of inner and outer worlds within the human being (Godwin, 1979).

Another Renaissance painter, Albrecht Curer, included the use of harmonic scales (Fischer, 1996b, pp. 37, 51) showing that the root harmonies of music, in keeping with Pythagorean concepts, correspond to good proportions in the human body. The idea of a correspondence between beauty as seen by the eye and harmony as heard by the ear begins to take on mystical proportions. Its relationship can be mathematically reproduced (Doczi, 1994, pp. 100–101). See Figure 3.4.

All parts of the human body share the same proportional limitations. The starting point unfolds at the center on top of the sacrum. Because of its central location in the body, the length of the top half and bottom half of the body are similar. The hand is a microcosmic mirror of the body, growing out of the wrist as the spine grows out of the sacrum. The relationship between hand to arm to trunk is also proportional, as is head to neck, trunk, legs, and feet. The graph illustrates the spread of approximations of human proportion to root harmonies found in music. Depicted are beautiful examples of

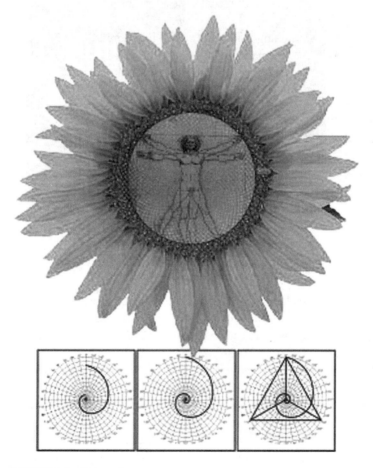

FIGURE 3.3   Human form.

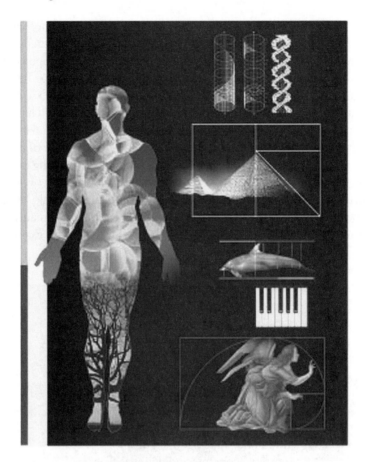

FIGURE 3.4   Human form and scale.

proportional harmonies found throughout the body, demonstrating that we have a harmonious presence in the universe.

Like a poised ballet dancer, our physical balancing center is located at the sacrum, while our spiritual center lies deep within our essential self. The potential for harmony and beauty exists within each person. The potential for disease and disorder is also possible.

The expert nurse can sense subtle shifts in delicate balance, hear a misalignment in the symphonic sounds of body breath, a disrupted rhythm of circulation. Before heralding signs are measurable, this artist senses a shift below the obvious, hears the unspoken against a background of silence, noting an asymmetrical shift from the normal patterns of health.

As well as its basic contribution to formation of pattern, the harmonies and rhythms of dinergy also form the basis for sharing, the art of living. Sharing is a condition of life, a generous act of grace that unites diversity in life-giving ways. Light, color, and sound, the artist's tools, share the same wave patterns and the same vibrational rates. The essence of all vibration and rhythm is a harmonious sharing of diversities—weak and strong, in and out, up and down, back and forth—at reoccurring time intervals. This oscillating pattern occurs in the tide of the ocean, in our heartbeats, in the creation of light and sound, in the growth of a plant.

Dancers share information, energy, and excitement, while friends share joys and concerns of the day. Shared stories and ideas in conversation, shared musical creation in song, shared worship in prayer, shared efforts towards problem resolution in community affairs, are part of everyday experience. The pattern of sharing is consistent in the birth of a phenomenon as well as throughout its dynamic growth and ultimate death. It emerges from a grateful heart. Albert Einstein observed that "A hundred times every day I remind myself that my inner and outer life depend on the labors of other men, living and dead, and that I must exert myself in order to give in the same measure as I have received and am still receiving" (Einstein, 1953, p. 1).

Many animal species model sharing in each other's distress while rescuing endangered community members. Biologist Edward Wilson noted that mutual aid and cooperation were an essential part of evolution, a precursor to all moral behavior (Wilson, 1980); sharing is creative. As we share with those who have less, we acquire more than if we had kept all the resources to ourselves.

Unfortunately, the materialistic drive in contemporary society finds the line between competition and shared cooperation sometimes difficult to distinguish. In terms of current economic and political policy, economist Barbara Ward observed, "When men or governments work intelligently and farsightedly for the good of others, they achieve their prosperity too . . . generosity is the best policy . . . our morals and our interest—seen in true perspective—do not pull us apart" (Ward, 1982, p. 150). Sharing as a basic pattern-forming process creates cooperation and abundance within a body, a group, and a civilization.

INTEGRATION: THE ART OF LIVING

Our continued development as a human species, and as a universe, is towards increasing capacity for goodness coupled with an innate drive for increasing intelligence—a journey towards beauty and wisdom. "Beauty is the harmony and concord of all parts, achieved in such a manner that nothing could be added or taken away or altered except for the worse" (Wittkower, 1992,

p. 33). History is filled with examples of too much leisure or luxury destroying our native beauty as well as it being destroyed by lack of life's basic necessities. Plato stated in his *Symposium,* that harmony and grace are born from the marriage of plenty and poverty. The pattern of sharing is a strong foundation that supports that which is beautiful and true to thrive in the world.

Our journey towards understanding is progressive, moving towards deeper levels of knowing. We begin as children with the accumulation of facts and data. School fills us with information designed to give us a basic understanding of the world in which we live. As we age, life experience becomes the teacher. An encounter with reality gives us lessons that go beyond what can be found in a book. We may get misinformation, but we do not have a misexperience. At some point in life, our worldview broadens and we begin to acquire knowledge, leading towards wisdom.

Wisdom and knowledge are the keys to turning mere survival into the art of living. Knowledge, like science, is a taking apart, while wisdom, a form of art, is a putting together. It synthesizes and integrates while knowledge analyzes and differentiates. Wisdom sees with eyes of mind, envisioning relation, wholeness, and unity. Knowledge accepts what can be verified by the senses, grasping the specific and the diverse. Both wisdom and knowledge are based on experience, but knowledge retains experience through the filter of conceptual thought, while wisdom speaks in images, symbols, and paradox. These two diversities complement each other in dinergistic style.

However, there are times when things come into our lives that do not fit any of the categories of thought; it is the presence of mystery. It can be a profound and disrupting experience such as illness, death, a sudden unplanned change. At other times, numinous feelings can arise from a simple, daily observation made with sacred eyes. It can emerge from seeing the perfect pattern of wholeness in a flower, smelling the air after a spring rain, or touching someone we love. In these extraordinary moments we converge with the hidden, harmonious nature that unites us as a universal family. In that space lies the possibility for expanding our awareness and consciousness.

When we share our own specific limitations with those of others in dinergistic fashion, we compliment each other's shortcomings and emerge a stronger, larger whole of a higher order. As an artist composing a life, we create living harmony comparable to the harmony found in the arts: music, dance, literature, and the sculpting of marble, wood, and clay.

Living in this fashion is our birthright; because nature's golden mean is part of the very fabric of our existence. The best human creations are timeless, ageless, and holy. They are beautiful and harmonious, and graciously generous. As we live in harmony with All-That-Is, we step into alignment with the flow of life in all of nature, and we are at one.

> *The only hope Mother Earth has for survival is our recovering creativity—*
> *which is of course, our divine power.*
> *Creativity is so satisfying, so important, not because it produces something*
> *but because the process is cosmological.*
> *There's joy and delight in giving birth.*
>
> Matthew Fox

BIBLIOGRAPHY

Abram, D. (1996). *The spell of the sensuous: Perception and language in a more-than-human world.* New York: Pantheon.

Chipp, H. B. (1956). *Theories of modern art.* Berkeley: University of California Press.

Doczi, G. (1994). *The power of limits: Proportional harmonies in nature, art and architecture.* Boston: Shambhala.

Dowson, R. (1979). *Art in its own terms.* New York: Taplinger.

Einstein, A. (1953). *The world as I see it.* New York: Oxford University Press.

Fischer, B. (1996a). *Man, grand reflection of the greater cosmos: Occult anatomy.* Vol. 1. Prescott, AZ: Subru.

Fischer, B. (1996b). *Pythagorean numerology: A summary of the esoteric properties of numbers.* Prescott, AZ: Clarity Works.

Godwin, J. (1979). *Robert Fludd.* Boulder, CO: Shambhala.

Kaku, M. (1994). *Hyperspace: A scientific odyssey through parallel universes, time warps, and the 10th dimension.* New York: Doubleday.

Leshan, L., & Margenau, H. (1982). *Einstein's space and Van Gogh's sky: Physical reality and beyond.* New York: Macmillan.

Pesut, D., & Herman, J. A. (1999). *Clinical reasoning: The art and science of critical and creative thinking.* Boston: Delmar.

Reed, L. (1968). *Art now.* London: Faber and Faber.

Russell, J. (1974). *The meanings of modern art.* New York: Harper and Row.

Glashow, S. (1988). *Interactions.* New York: Warner.

Shlain, L. (1991). *Art and physics: Parallel visions in space, time and light.* New York: Quill.

Steiner, R. (2001). *The fourth dimension: Sacred geometry, alchemy and mathematics.* Great Barrington: Anthroposophic Press.

Ward, B. (1982). *The rich nations and the poor nations.* New York: W. W. Norton.

Wilson, E. (1980). *Sociobiology: The abridged edition.* Cambridge, MA: Harvard University Press.

Wittkower, R. (1992). *Architectural principles in the age of humanism.* London: Alec Tiranti.

CHAPTER 4

The Human Essence

Unfolding Inner Potential

Within each individual on this large and complicated world there lives an astonishing potential of greatness. Yet it is rare that these hidden gifts are brought to life unless by chance of fate or commitment to inner growth.

Unknown teacher

We stand poised on the threshold of human history where humanity is on the brink of a new understanding regarding the true depth of our human potential. Alienation and hatred are part of the ongoing saga of war and terrorism, reminding us of the depths to which we can plunge when fear and anger rule. At the same time, we see reflections of the best of human nature in the demonstrated love and heroism that depict a greater humanity.

We can explore the rich journey of the universe across time from multiple perspectives including science, religion, philosophy, literature, and the arts. As we walk with our ancestors, we see the result of forces acting upon them many millennia ago. What becomes clear is the fact that what we will be tomorrow depends on our present choices, choices strongly influenced by a number of constraints that are part of the evolutionary makeup of humanity.

Our unfolding story is influenced by the genes that make up the human body, by instincts that trigger an action below the level of conscious awareness. Choices are strongly influenced by cultural heritage, the systems that code appropriate behavior, often limiting us to conduct better suited to some past time. And then there is the belief system of religion that fosters intolerance of others who are not members. Recognition of the forces and choices that limit our journey towards increasing consciousness and human capacity makes it possible to become liberated from them (Csikszentmihalyi, 1993).

A new urgency is felt in our continuing search for self-awareness. For the past 400 years the world of science has given us discoveries that would have amazed our ancestors. It has explained the birth of the universe from a tiny seed to a self-expanding cosmos and provided images of immense galaxies and subatomic quarks. But science alone cannot provide what we need today, for we are now moving beyond our physical existence in the external world into an equally daring and disciplined exploration of our inner life. The threshold we are crossing moves us into the landscape of the soul and transcendence, leading to personal and global transformation.

As we review the unfolding history of human potential, the evolution of human capacity from a tiny cell to spectacular new abilities and levels of experience becomes evident. Humankind's exploration of the inner life is uncovering new frontiers of creativity that are antidotes for the hatred and alienation that has plagued us for so long. It heralds the dawn of a cultural transformation beyond anything we have heretofore imagined.

OUR BEGINNINGS: A SLOW AND SOLITARY JOURNEY

In his compelling book, *A Brief History of Everything,* Ken Wilbur observes that "There is a common evolutionary thread running from matter to life to mind. Certain common patterns, or laws, or habits keep repeating themselves in all those domains" (Wilber, 1996, p. 19). He suggests that, according to the world's great wisdom traditions, looking at those extraordinary patterns reveal the unfolding of *Spirit-in-action.* Every stage of development finds consciousness manifesting and realizing more of itself, recognizing more of its own true nature.

Stages of higher development modeled by ancient teachers and adepts reflect our own deep potential. Looking carefully at these lives in light of our own continuing emergence informs us about what personal and collective evolution has in store for us tomorrow. This helps us make concrete sense of the experiences and observations that comprise our own path towards wholeness. As we identify and practice new ways of being, we are transformed.

Great debate exists within the scientific, philosophical, and religious worlds regarding the theory of evolution. The facts demonstrating our continuing development and advancement as a universe, a civilization, as individuals, are everywhere noted (Berry & Swimme, 1992; Kaufman, 1995; Lloyd, 1923). In spite of growing evidence, some people still deny its existence. "One cause of such misunderstanding is a failure to distinguish evolution as fact from theories on how and why it is happening" (Redfield & Murphy, 2002, p. 73).

However explained and understood, the meandering course of evolution from the beginning of the universe, to the appearance of living species, and the emergence of humanity has created the inorganic, biological, and human worlds. In this pattern we can see that even the process of evolution has evolved. The underlying pattern of this ever-evolving universe is movement to ever greater complexities in the material world and the growing capacities of humanity.

The appearance of plant life and the emergence of humanity marked the beginnings of two new evolution eras; these were moments of evolutionary transcendence (Pearce, 2002). Quantum shifts of this magnitude were made possible through the countless changes in complexity that preceded them. Evolutionary theorist Stebbins (1969) noted that approximately 640 thousand small steps in organic evolution resulted in less than 100 major changes in plant and animal development during hundreds of millions of years of evolutionary progress.

Humankind has followed the same prefigured design in our development across time. Patterns and trends suggest that we are approaching an emerging evolutionary domain similar to the epic shift from inorganic to plant life or the emergence of human form. The convergence of the birth of spiritual awareness among our ancestors and the recent scientific discoveries about the untapped capacities for life are potentiating a shift of unprecedented nature.

Evolution began accelerating our human journey with the convergence of intelligence, communication, and domestic skills. Our species began to form creative social groups, harness fire, develop tools, form words, communicate, and create art forms. In the Stone Age our evolutionary journey was launched as we continued our efforts to make sense of the world in which we live.

At one point these ancestors began to develop markedly beyond the capacity of their forbearers. *Shamans* were centrally involved in this acceleration of human development in various roles such as medicine men and women, masters of ritual, artists, and guides to worlds beyond the senses. Shamans have long been the primary mediators within their communities while also offering contact with the spirit world. While they were expert at healing and assisting with love and battle, their greatest contribution was in their capacity for altered states of consciousness used in healing, dream interpretation, and bringing the community closer to other worlds.

Studies in the Americas, Siberia, Central Asia, and Australia show remarkable similarities between shamanic practices worldwide. Most Stone-Age cultures believed that a shaman in trance would transverse other worlds to assist with their activities around healing physical and spiritual ailments and better preside over rites of passage such as marriage, birth, and death. Shamanism was the first institutionalization of visions and practices that opened extraordinary powers to contact the Transcendent. They were the forerunners of the prophets, saints, and seers of the world's great religions (Harner, 1990).

SHARING THE PATH: A CONVERGENCE OF COLLECTIVES

Thousands of years after the appearance of shamanism, the birth of *mystery schools* appeared in Greece, Syria, Anatolia, Egypt, and Persia. They involved similar activities, including adoration of a specific deity, rites of spiritual transformation, and very elaborate religious rituals and dramas. These rituals and teachings fostered an intuitive sense that the soul is secretly connected with the divine, pointing countless people towards a greater life to come (Hall, 1986; Meyer, 1987).

During the second millennium B.C.E., another significant step in human consciousness occurred in India with the emergence of the *Vedic* culture. The oldest collection of religious texts used today, they are divided into four bodies: hymns, prayers, rites, and healing practices; mythologies of ancient India; spiritual philosophy; and instructions for yoga practices. These were developed to put these teachings into the hands of the people, literally allowing them to "sit at the feet of the masters" (Pannikar, 1977).

Between the seventh and fourth centuries B.C.E. in the Middle East, Asia, and Greece another spiritual awakening occurred, referred to as the "Axial Age" because of its impact on people living in one half of the world. China experienced the emergence of Taoism while Greece and Athens experienced the awakening of philosophy. The Jews were guided by great prophets, while India was incorporating the teachings of Buddha. The countless insights from this era seeded the beginnings of the evolutionary leap we are about to take today.

The *Tao Te Ching*, written by Lao-Tzu in the sixth century B.C.E., articulated the convergence of Chinese philosophy and shamanism. It gave rise to: metaphysical teachings; the practice of feng shui, which helps landscaping lie in accord with natural contours and forces; calligraphy, which calls for the student to trust the hand's instinctive flow; acupuncture, herbal medicines, and tai chi, all of which are based on movements that harmonize the body with the energy of *chi*; and Taoist art, including the yin-yang symbol widely used today. More than any sacred tradition before or since, Taoism supports a philosophy and set of practices that promote aesthetic harmony with all that is (Lao-Tzu, 1992, 2001).

In the fifth century B.C.E., *Buddhism* was the reforming religious culture in India, which remains the primary laboratory and disseminator of this philosophy today. Gautama Buddha, the founder, identified "four noble truths." The first states that all life is marked by suffering; the second notes that suffering is caused by desire; the third states that there is release from suffering by blowing out the flames of desire; and, the fourth highlights the way to nirvana via the eightfold noble path. This path includes right understanding, right thought, right speech, right action, right livelihood, right effort, right concentration, and right mindfulness (Armstrong, 2001).

This spiritual tradition stresses commitment to ideas and the practice of disciplines that can produce freedom from suffering while promoting spiritual understanding through detachment and the acquisition of wisdom. A primary tenet of the belief system is a powerful ethic of service to those in need. The spirit of compassion is a foundational principle in the doctrine of the bodhisattva. Within this tradition is a vast information store regarding human development that is essential as the world becomes increasingly complex. Its power lies in the integration of Taoist, Shaman, Zen, and other practices into its roots within the yogas of ancient India (Hahn, 1999).

In making these cultural adaptations, Buddhism has transcended the insights of its founder and early practitioners, becoming a great repository of liberating practices that can transform our potential, including meditation, visualization, energy mobilization, and mindfulness training. Its greatest power lies in its learned ability to adapt these transformative disciplines to the various cultures in order to enhance their adoption. As we move more towards our emergent nature, our understanding will increasingly incorporate some of these practices.

While the East was moving in this direction, Greek city-states began to emerge on the Mediterranean Sea. The seeds of Western culture were planted, with developments in mathematics and discoveries in the physical world; with the unfolding of rhetoric and philosophy; and with a blending of history, art, and politics that gave rise to individual rights.

One of Greece's greatest gifts, however, was fostered with the presence of Plato and Socrates. These physically and spiritually vigorous men, through their *philosophical dialogue and rhetoric,* gave birth to the capacity for self-reflection and self-understanding. Living from 470–399 B.C.E., Socrates was a prominent critic of conventional opinion. His liberating skepticism questioned conventional assumptions about the world, and he declared that the unexamined life was not worth living (Guthrie, 1960). He stimulated self-inquiry and examination of social norms, and established the Socratic method of inquiry, which has inspired ethical integrity for several millennia.

His famous student, Plato, became a great philosopher who explored timeless questions regarding identity and the ways we acquire knowledge. He examined practical ways to live a good life, and to improve education and social politics. He founded "The Academy" on his family's land, which flourished for 900 years. At this place students were guided to find the true, the good, and the beautiful through practiced acts of contemplation, discourse, and moral behavior.

Both men brought an unprecedented intellectual range and flexibility, integrating the physical, social, moral, and spiritual worlds of their time. Aristotle, Plato's greatest student, took their work to another level when he developed his theory of forms, holding that eternal ideas corresponded with humanities less-than-perfect efforts. He was the founder of classification systems, setting standards that later established the field of biology. His work would be pivotal in guiding Charles Darwin's evolutionary theory many years later.

The cumulative work of these early intellectual explorers influenced subsequent Jewish, Christian, and Islamic philosophy and practice. These *courageous pioneers of the integral spirit* showed the world how to join together seemingly unrelated functions of social understanding, philosophical speculation, mystical insight, and the individual practice of virtue. Their playful, fertile, and creative experimentation laid the groundwork for the intellectual flexibility and individual morality of future generations, including our own (Plato, 1928).

The Axial Age was also influenced by the great *Jewish Prophets*, Isaiah, Micah, Amos, Jeremiah, and Elijah, who lived between the ninth and fourth centuries B.C.E. They broadened the tribal view of Yahweh (the Hebrew name for God), making him a God for all people. They reinforced the notion that all men and women, including the sick and disadvantaged, were equally children of this living God. They underscored the need for ethical standards if people are to live peacefully together. And, they set the stage for religion to become a strong political force (Heschel, 1956).

One of the greatest contributions of the Jewish age was their emphasis on life as a journey towards better things. It was a sharp break from the cyclical nature of life as proposed by Eastern and Greek belief systems. Jewish life was viewed as a mystical practice leading towards union with God. Such a life required social justice and nonviolence, universal love and forgiveness, and a life of active service to the less fortunate. Many of these tenets would later influence Martin Buber and other contemporary psychologists.

Several centuries later, another Jewish prophet emerged, Jesus of Nazareth. Six hundred years before he appeared the Jews had begun to look for a Messiah; many inside and outside of the Jewish faith identified Jesus as this Messiah. Within 300 years of Jesus's death, *Christianity* had become the dominant religion of the Roman Empire, and in the two millennia since, it has become the most popular religion on earth. The principal message of this belief system is the necessity of letting God's love for humanity flow from ourselves to others, even those who attack us. It is a message of unconditional love, Christian fellowship with others, and a life of compassion, forgiveness, and service. By embodying Jesus's teaching that God's love channeled through us can save the world, we develop our capacities for transformation and further spiritual advance (Stephen, 1999).

Islam is the second most popular and the fastest-growing world religion today. With roots in Abraham, it moved through Judaism and Christianity, only to be redefined by Muhammad, who felt the message of these religions was too distorted. Devotional practices, including prayer five times daily, demonstrate a commitment to God. Three blessings are given, thru *Sufism,* to those who love God with devotion: submission, faith, and an abiding aware- ness of God. The quest for a direct experience of God is both the crown of religious life and the path towards truth (Nicholson, 1967).

Since the mid-twentieth century, Sufism has been growing in Europe and America among people seeking authentic spiritual realization that transcends monasticism. Many teachers, such as Gurdjieff (Fisher, 1996), have inspired groups devoted to meditation, self-inquiry, and devotional exercises devel- oped in esoteric Sufi schools. Although Islam, like many religions, has bred dogmatism and intolerance, it also has elevated the moral and spiritual lives of people worldwide.

Expanding Understanding: Movement From Religious to Secular

The movement of the *Renaissance* flourished during Europe's Middle Ages. This period of rebirth was a precursor to the Modern Age. An era of un- precedented development spanned the arenas of art and science, religion and philosophy, architecture and social systems. However, it did not resolve the great suffering of the masses, as war and poverty spawned by the Crusades and the decline of the Greco-Roman empire continued a caste system of government (Tarnas, 1991).

Leonardo Da Vinci embodied the ideal Renaissance personality: a self- described disciple of experiment. His work was infused with great originality that focused on problems of science and society, with notable outcomes in the design of buildings and machines, weapons of war, and works of art. Simultaneously, as great scientists' and artists' creativity overflowed, the turn- ing towards supernatural beliefs of the past era was increasingly replaced by the worldly realism of emerging science and the affirmation of the individual. The Renaissance was an era whose emphasis was on human expression, power, and fulfillment, and the embracing of discoveries, inventions, and insights birthed in an atmosphere committed to the love of learning and creativity (Leonardo Da Vinci, 1956).

As the eighteenth century began, the focus on humanity and nature had moved westward. It was kindled by freedom of expression with speech and pen. Increasingly frequent and direct communication, coupled with the use of reason, and a revolt against religious oppression or the rule of kings, fostered stunning advances in science and technology. Those seeking truth were searching for a clarifying and unifying vision to transcend the destructive religious conflicts of the day. This quest gave birth to the *Scientific Revolution* and the *Enlightenment*.

In the light of increasing scientific discovery, supernatural explanations were no longer needed to explain the world and human nature. The ensuing literary, scientific, and philosophical movements among notables such as Copernicus, Galileo, Newton, and other scientists, along with Descartes, Locke, Hume, and other thinkers, built on their rich past while challenging traditional wisdom. The call went out for intellectual liberty, the emergence of reason, and the testing and validating of the irrefutable laws of science (Kuhn, 1970).

While science was progressive, its shadow side began to emerge. Scientists increasingly rejected the findings of contemplatives as science increasingly turning away from nonconfirmable facts of the inner life. Many also began to reject all spiritual phenomena, giving rise to a strictly materialistic view of the world and humankind. Along with the liberation of the human spirit and overthrow of despotic regimes, the use and abuse of science also contributed to the exploitation and destruction of the earth and the natural world—a trend that continues.

As we review the great human journey, the story reveals a greater life pressing to be born within humanity. We see that as certain practices are incorporated into daily life, enlarging capacities can be nurtured and eventually integrated as a permanent aspect of our being. We also develop an appreciation for the fundamental social forces that work against them.

As people, we are seeking for a worldview that gives both context and guidance to our quest to transcend the dogma and superstition that has for so long divided us. Contemporary spiritual leaders such as Vietnamese Buddhist monk Thich Nhat Hahn have observed that the next Buddha will not appear in the form of an individual. Instead the new spiritually centered force will emerge in the form of a community of people living in loving-kindness and mindful awareness (Pearce, 2002). Nursing holds the potential for serving society in this capacity today.

THE POSSIBLE HUMAN: A BIOLOGY OF TRANSCENDENCE

Since the beginning of the early nineteenth century, both scholars and scientists have unearthed a wide range of discoveries to create the largest body of knowledge ever available on the extraordinary capacity of human functioning. Coupled with increasing access to wisdom literature translated into multiple languages, there has emerged a vast array of educational and therapeutic experiments, and countless empirical studies on human capacity, the range and creativity of which is breathtaking in its scope.

Transcendence implies the ability to rise beyond. There is a bitter irony in the fact that we have a history so rich in lofty philosophy and noble ideas, and yet are experiencing a degree of violence unprecedented in human history. New studies demonstrate that neither our violence nor our capacity for transcendence is specifically a moral/ethical issue. Rather, it is primarily a biological one (Pearce, 2004, pp. 27–32).

Our history of behavior has derailed our personal development of biological capacities for transcendence. We continue to project the bad that is out there towards each other, while the good is transferred to the wise and sage among us. A new breed of biologists and neuroscientists has uncovered the root to our paradoxical behavior of feeling one thing, saying another, and acting from an impulse different than either.

These new scientists have discovered that we have five different neural structures, or brains, within us. Four of the five lie within our head, representing the whole evolution of life preceding us: reptilian, old mammalian, new mammalian, and human. Each new structure emerged to offer us the possibility of going beyond former behavior, while simultaneously creating new problems for us to solve.

The fifth brain of our system lies in our heart, just as poets have long believed. The new field of neurocardiology has uncovered this brain center in our heart, which functions in a dynamic way with the fourfold brain in our head. This head-heart dynamic affects, reflects, and determines our responsiveness outside the field of our conscious awareness. As we become more aware of nature's head-heart dynamic we begin to cooperate with this mutually interdependent spirit and the activity between our intelligence and our intellect, our biology and our spirit. The unification and transcendence of our splintered selves may be the next intelligent evolutionary shift.

The pathbreaking studies of leading neuroscientist Paul MacLean span more than six decades and give a clear map of three neural systems in our head and the parallel connection to three major evolutionary periods in the universe: reptilian, old mammalian, and new mammalian. Each neural system carries a blueprint of potential intelligences, abilities, and capabilities developed during each epoch (MacLean, 1993).

Nature never abandons a working system, but instead enlarges and expands the old to increase efficiency. Each new evolutionary brain was established to solve a challenge in our ever-changing environment. When each gets integrated into the other our capacity increases tenfold. However, when integration fails, we become a house divided against itself, with great inner (and outer) conflict the result.

Our *hindbrain,* the reptilian brain, is the oldest member, whose primary function is giving us awareness of the outer sensory world. Comprised of the sensory-motor system, the spinal cord, and a vast network of neural connections, this process functions well below our level of awareness. It manages our physical well-being by controlling basic physiological activity. It functions in a very habitual, patterned way and cannot alter its inherited or learned patterns of behavior.

Originally designed to elude predators, this oldest structure is highly skilled at deceptive procedures. It helps us to be multifaceted when threatened and can be used, in conjunction with our higher neocortex, to rationalize and justify morally deceptive behavior.

This brain registers present tense only. In emergencies, its reflexive system can alert the neocortex to mobilize all systems for body defense. Emotion has no impact on this center, so clarity and swiftness are its hallmarks. However, there is an interpreter mode between this brain and the neocortex that passes through our emotional-cognitive system upon command. This broader connection allows for the neocortex to stand back and moderate or redirect a sensory report, minimizing what at times could be a violent reaction from the predatory nature of this brain center.

The second brain to emerge in humankind was the old mammalian, *limbic,* or emotional-cognitive brain. Here nature added to the limited reptilian senses the extraordinary senses of smell and hearing, which opened up a whole new world of higher order for the sensory system. As the seat of learning and memory, this space is encoded with multiple functions and behaviors, which includes a mothering capacity to serve as the limbic function for an infant until this aspect of its brain is fully developed at the age of three.

This nurturing emotional brain computes a past and present state and serves as the foundation for relationships. It gives us an awareness of our interior subjective world along with our feelings concerning the outer world and our relationship with it. Emotions are the collective tools we utilize to qualitatively evaluate our relationships, facilitating an association to the world as a sophisticated object standing outside of it, rather than from a simple reflexive act.

The newer mammalian brain or *neocortex* serves as our verbal-intellectual brain. This brain possesses the awareness of past, present, and future. It introduces language and thinking, the capacity to observe all factors in a situation rather than react from instinct alone. This high brain is five times larger than the other two combined, hosting a hundred billion neurons, each capable of interacting with a hundred thousand others to create fields of coordinated action. Neural fields constantly shift and change to update their intelligence reports, translating external information and data into thought and imagination within.

Evolution opened an entirely new universe with the gift of awareness embedded in the neocortex. With a capacity to predict the future, problem solving became a human potential. The high brain also holds an impulse towards novelty that fosters creative imagination, our highest human capacity (Steiner, 1969).

Brain development occurs in a nested hierarchy, beginning with the reptilian brain in the first trimester of pregnancy, followed by the old mammalian in the second trimester, and the new mammalian brain in the third. A new fourth brain makes its entrance after birth. What makes each of these evolving neural systems uniquely human is the overall context into which they are placed, each articulating with the other while holding limitless capacity for network development with similar fields.

Bruce Lipton, a cellular biologist (Lipton & Bertsch, 1991), demonstrated how the first cell created is a template for all subsequent cellular development. The essential nature of any system is that it maintains its integrity while playing a new and expanded role in partnership with emerging new structures. In a two-way exchange each cell and each brain modifies the other to some degree. The resulting movement beyond limitations, the hallmark of transcendence, is not reached at the expense of any other system. This facilitates a sustaining field for all involved.

Whether we live a life of creative adventure or close ourselves in a defensive way depends to a large extent upon the first years of life when the new fourth brain, the *prefrontal cortex,* emerges to support our higher intellect (Ferris, 1992). This most recent and largest brain addition resides in the ridge of our brow. Functions attributed to it include the higher human virtues of love, compassion, empathy, and understanding as well as advanced intellectual skills. It is considered to house the seat of higher intellect: our ability to compute, reason and analyze, and think creatively. It also includes our ability to regulate emotions, control our impulses, and modify reflexive behavior; in other words, it governs the activity of the other three brains in civilized fashion (Jerison, 1997).

Schore's prolific work in this area shows that development of the prefrontal lobes is experience-dependent; the environment must provide appropriate stimuli if full growth is to occur. First stage of growth occurs within the first year of life, and again in mid-adolescence if adequate affirmation in a positive environment is experienced. Full development occurs around the age of 21, with yet another chance for transcendence at approximately age 30 (Schore, 1994).

If life is filled with fear, violence, shaming, rules, and other emotionally depleting activities such as stress and anxiety within the mother or the environment, the prefrontal lobes decline. Nurturing an infant induces long-lasting changes in the adult frontal cortex, leading to permanent modifications that increase exploratory behavior and playfulness, important roles in regulating higher-order information processing.

Failure to nurture leads to increasing inability of young people to modify primitive impulses and behaviors as this coordinating function is diminished. Statistics from 1995 indicate that on average, every day in America, 18 children were shot by other children. As of 2000, suicide became the third leading cause of death in children between ages 5 and 17. Continued exposure to violence in music and film, guns and police protection in the school systems, terrorism in the news, and an endless string of "no" and "don't" must be vigorously offset with an emphasis on the nurturance and love of infants and adolescents if this alarming trend is to be reversed (Pearce, 2004, p. 148).

Six decades ago cellular research led to the discovery that alters not only the way we view the heart but also our relationship to the universe. The discovery of the triune heart—electromagnetic, neural, and hormonal in nature—fostered a new field of medicine, neuro-cardiology (Armour & Ardell, 1994). While all living forms produce an electrical charge, the heart cell has an electrical output 40 to 60 times greater than a brain wave. This energy forms an electromagnetic field that extends 12 to 15 feet beyond our body, its greatest strength residing in the first three feet.

The traditional view of the heart as a pump is enriched when examined from the perspective of the triune heart, where the pumping function is enhanced by the synchronistic contraction and expansion of the blood vessels themselves, the motility and plasticity of blood cells that change shape according to the size of vessel they are moving through, contraction of the skeletal muscles, and the flow of blood in spiral-like vortices from grooves built into the blood vessels themselves. As blood dashes into the heart chamber from an open heart valve, the rush of swirling blood forms a vortex, adding to its electromagnetic field (Marinelli, 1995). See Figure 4.1.

The force of this electromagnetic field produces a donut-shaped torus, much as magnets create an arc from filings placed within their field. The axis of this torus extends from the pelvic floor to the top of the skull. Comprised of an organic and living force, the torus is a very stable energy field that tends to self-perpetuate. Scientists conjecture that all energy systems, from the smallest atomic field to the largest universal level, are toroid in form. This leads to speculation that there is one universal torus that encompasses an infinite number of interacting, holographic tori within its spectrum (Childre, 1999).

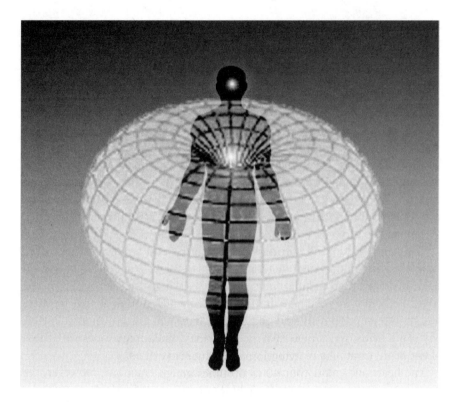

FIGURE 4.1   The heart's torus.

Our solar system, with the sun at center, is also toroidal in nature. Fluctuations within its energy field impact all others through the corresponding magnetic lines of earth. We exist in a nested hierarchy of toroid energy systems, making each of us as much the center of the universe as any other point or creature. Because these electromagnetic fields are holographic in nature, this gives us equal access to all that exists (Greene, 1999).

Producing energy is the first characteristic of the triune heart. Neurotransmitters, the second trait, create the "brain in the heart" as over half of the cardiac cells are comprised of neurons, clustered into ganglia similar to those found in the brain. One aggregate of the heart's neural ganglia is scattered throughout body tissue, muscle spindles, and organs through a connection to the spinal cord and peripheral neuron system. A second grouping has direct and unmediated connection with the emotional limbic brain, fostering an ongoing dialogue between heart and brain.

In embryonic and fetal development, a rudimentary human heart comes first, followed by the formation of the brain, and then the body. Before becoming a four-chambered heart, the rudimentary heart furnishes the electromagnetic (em) field, which envelops the embryo from its inception. This em field is surrounded by the mother's more powerful heart energy, stabilizing the infant's heart field as it takes on the imprint of the mother.

The third influencer of the heart on the brain is hormonal in nature, resulting in the conclusion that the heart is an endocrine gland (Raloff, 1998). The atrium of the heart produces the hormone ANF, which can influence and modulate the emotional-cognitive system of the brain. Other heart-generated hormones have also been uncovered, including tranquilizers that keep us in balance and harmony with each other and the earth. Because the heart is connected to every facet of both the body and the brain, it is the intellect of the heart, not the brain that must coordinate the signals from the pancreas, liver, spleen, and so on.

The heart, earth, and sun provide the earth's electromagnetic spectrum, supplying the fundamental materials for creating our reality. Our heart's em field shields us from inappropriate frequencies while also selecting, from the larger hologram in which we are nested, frequency groupings that facilitate our growth, development, and ongoing life. Through this holographic hierarchy of em fields, we can modulate our heart and brain frequencies with those of the earth, creating a reciprocal relationship between us.

The heart and mind connection speaks through emotions. However, the heart has no neural structures to perceive or analyze the context, nature, details, or logic of our emotional reports. The heart is unable to judge the validity of these reports, so it responds to them as basic facts. A state of harmony and love connects us to the high cortical areas where creativity and problem solving reside. If the message is negative, the heart makes an adaptive shift from the slower reflective intellect (slow thoughts) of the frontal lobes and neocortex to the swift reptilian brain (fast thoughts) linked with the emotional brain, where survival memories and maneuvers reside.

This sudden shift from forebrain to hindbrain is not voluntary; it occurs outside of our awareness. In this archaic and defensive mind-set we have limited access to our intellectual capacity, falling back on our defenses or revenge strategies. These ancient patterns are supported by powerful field energies of consensual reality; group mind-set, and crowd comfort. These fields are constantly reinforced through much of the information and activity occurring in the mass culture in which we reside. We pick up that vibrational energy as surely as we respond to our own, unless there is a conscious effort to detach from it.

Our emerging potential cannot be utilized, nor can our dilemma get resolved by intellect or ethical efforts alone. The hope for transcendence lies in our ability to break from the mass mind-set, and turn to our heart. The minute we recognize that a stressful event is forming, we can shift our focus from the threat to our heart. Recalling an event infused with love and gratitude immediately blocks the automatic negative reaction to a stressful event. From this quiet and centered place we can hear the wisdom of our heart and body-mind, selecting options that move towards our well-being as well as that of the world. At each moment we must open ourselves again and again, making each decision through this new intelligence until, at last, we have shifted the focal point of our response to life into the transcendent realm of active intelligence. This begins our true healing journey.

Someday, after mastering winds, waves, tides and gravity,
We shall harness the energy of love,
And for the second time in the history of the world,
Man will have discovered fire.

Pierre Teilhard De Chardin

BIBLIOGRAPHY

Armour, J. A., & Ardell, J. (Eds.) (1994). *Neurocardiology.* New York: Oxford University Press.

Armstrong, K. (2001). *Buddha.* San Francisco: HarperCollins.

Berry, T., & Swimme, B. (1992). *The universe story.* San Francisco: Harper and Row.

Childre, L. (1999). *The HeartMath solution.* San Francisco: HarperSanFrancisco.

Csikszentmihalyi, M. (1993). *The evolving self: A psychology for the third millennium.* New York: Harper Collins.

Ferris, T. (1992). *The mind's sky: Human intelligence in a cosmic context.* New York: Bantam.

Fisher, B. S. (1996). *The Gurdjieff teachings: A compilation and summary.* Prescott, AZ: Subru.

Greene, B. (1999). *The elegant universe: Superstrings, hidden dimensions and the quest for the ultimate theory.* New York: Random House.

Guthrie, W.K.C. (1960). *The Greek philosophers: From Thales to Aristotle.* San Francisco: HarperCollins.

Hahn, T. N. (1999). *The heart of Buddha's teaching: Transforming suffering into peace, joy and liberation.* New York: Broadway Books.

Hall, B. P. (1986). *The genesis effect.* New York: Paulist Press.

Harner, M. (1990). *The way of the shaman.* New York: HarperCollins.

Heschel, A. (1956). *God in search of man.* New York: Jewish Publication Society.

Jerison, H. J. (1997). Evolution of prefrontal cortex. In N. A. Krasnegor (Ed.), *Development of the prefrontal cortex: Evolution, neurobiology and behavior* (pp. 118–126). Baltimore, MD: Paul H. Brookes.

Kaufman, S. (1995). *At home in the universe.* Oxford: Oxford University Press.

Kuhn, T. (1970). *The structure of the scientific revolution* (2nd edition). Chicago: University of Chicago Press.

Lao-Tzu. (1992). *Tao Te Ching: A new English version* (S. Mitchell, Trans.). San Francisco: HarperCollins.

Lao-Tzu. (2001). *Tao Te Ching: The definitive edition* (J. Star, Trans.). New York: Tarcher/Putnam.

Lipton, B. H., & Bertsch, K. G. (1991). Microvessel endothelial cell transdifferentiation: Phenotypic characterization. *Differentiation, 46,* 117–133.

Lloyd, M. C. (1923). *Emergent evolution.* New York: Holt and Company.

MacLean, P. (1993). The brain and subjective experience: Question of multilevel role of resonance. *Journal of Mind and Behavior, 18*(2–3), 247–268.

Marinelli, R. (1995, Fall/Winter). The heart is not a pump: A refutation of the pressure propulsion premise of heart function. *Frontier Perspectives, 5*(1), 91–97.

Meyer, M. (1987). *The ancient mysteries: A sourcebook of sacred texts of the mystery religion of the ancient Mediterranean world.* San Francisco: HarperCollins.

Nichodemi, G., et al. (Eds.). (1956). *Leonardo Da Vinci* by Leonardo Da Vinci. London: Reynal, Williams and Morrow.

Nicholson, R. (1967). *Studies in Islamic mysticism.* Cambridge: Cambridge University Press. (Reprint of 1921 edition: *The idea of personality in Sufism.* Cambridge: Cambridge University Press.)

Pannikar, R. (1977). *The Vedic experience: Mantramanjari.* Berkeley: University of California Press.

Pearce, J. C. (2002). *The biology of transcendence.* Rochester, VT: Park Street Press.

Plato. (1928). *Symposium* (A. Niehamas and P. Woodruff, Trans.). Oxford: Oxford University Press.

Raloff, J. (1998, February). EMF's biological influences: Electromagnetic fields exert effects on and through hormones. *Science News, 153,* 154.

Redfield, J., & Murphy, M. (2002). *God and the evolving universe: The next steps in personal evolution.* New York: Jeremy P. Tarcher/Putnum.

Schore, A. N. (1994). *Affect regulation and the origin of the self: The neurobiology of emotional development.* Hillsdale, NJ: Lawrence Erlbaum Associates.

Stebbins, G. I. (1969). *The basis of progressive evolution.* Charlotte: University of North Carolina Press.

Steiner, R. (1969). *Knowledge of the higher worlds and their attainment.* London: Steiner.

Stephen, M. (1999). *The gospel according to Jesus: A new translation and guide to his essential teaching for believers and unbelievers.* San Francisco: HarperCollins.

Tarnas, R. (1991). *The passion of the Western mind: Understanding the ideas that have shaped our worldview.* San Francisco: Harmony.

Wilber, K. (1996). *A brief history of everything.* Boston: Shambhala.

SECTION III

A Healing Presence:
The Power of One

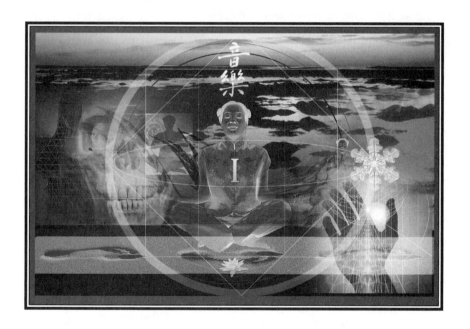

*Good listening is ultimately a form
of love. When we listen well we
not only celebrate the other
but we also celebrate ourselves.
By sharing our presence with reverence
we re-enchant and resacralize the world.*

Unknown teacher

CHAPTER 5

Vibrant Health

The Path of Balance

The body is the visible soul,
and the soul is the invisible body.
The body and soul are not divided anywhere,
they are parts of each other,
they are parts of One Whole.

Osho

$\mathbf{A}$s a vibrant, living field of energy, each being touches, and is touched by, All-That-Is. Energies from the sun and earth flow through every cell, in-forming our body and our health. As a distinct self-regulating universe, our body occupies—uniquely—a space in the cosmos; we are a force in this world.

Most current approaches to health stem from the Newtonian viewpoint that the human body is a complex machine. Expanding our worldview to the Einsteinian physics perspective, we see the human being as a multidimensional organism, comprised of physical cellular systems, in dynamic exchange with complex and diverse regulatory energetic fields. In this vibrant and dynamic world, health and healing also includes influencing the subtle energy fields surrounding the body instead of simply manipulating the cells and organs with drugs and surgery. The belief that we are frail biochemical machines controlled by genes is being usurped by the knowledge that we are powerful creators of our lives and the world in which we live.

HEALTH BELIEFS: LIVING OUR DEFINITIONS

How do you define health—and illness? Our beliefs and definitions guide our nursing practice. If health is the absence of disease we approach the patient with an arsenal of weapons to conquer the body invaders in warrior fashion. If, on the other hand, it is about balance in multiple dimensions of being, the approach seeks to restore what is innately within and around the individual being supported. Becoming clear about our own health beliefs is the first step to actualizing our professional accountability to others.

In a linear and dualistic world, health is viewed as the absence of disease. This pervading worldview treats health as a commodity that we can acquire if perfect self-control is maintained. We tend to judge those who are considered less diligent in their health practices, including ourselves. In such a world, war is waged on things that threaten the body. Like the surgical bombing carried out during the Persian Gulf War, we attack the invader with antibiotics to kill it, surgery to remove it, or radiation to destroy it.

There is a decided value of good for health, while illness is seen as bad and undesirable. Healing practices are prescribed. The healer knows what is best, labeling the patient noncompliant if orders are not obeyed. This model of practice has been carried out for hundreds of years. However, a new paradigm for health is emerging; one asserting that *disease is a manifestation of health* (Newman, 1986).

The theory of complimentarity states that two opposites, in relationship, create a whole. Quantum physicist David Bohm observed:

> When you trace a particular absolute notion to what appears to be its logical conclusion, you find it to be identical with its opposite, and therefore the whole dualism collapses. Reason first shows you that opposites pass into each other, and then you discover that one opposite reflects the other, and finally, you find that they are identical to each other—not really different at all. (Bohm, 1980, p. 39)

Our journey across the life span is a movement towards authenticity, peace, and community. As nurse theorist Margaret Newman helped her mother navigate through a terminal illness she noticed something intriguing: the more debilitated her mother became, the more she experienced wholeness and peacefulness. Years later that observation matured into her theory called "Health as Expanding Consciousness": Health is an ever-increasing awareness of ourselves and who we are in relation to life in all its fullness, an unfolding of our essence and our destiny (Newman, 1986, p. 37).

Newman believes that health is the expansion of consciousness that transcends the illness-wellness dichotomy. In this world, disease fosters the chaotic energy breakdown that allows for integration and movement towards new order. The nurse assists with pattern recognition, and through a therapeutic but nonintervention-focused relationship, assists the person in gaining new awareness that facilitates an enlarged perspective on life.

Another nursing theorist, Dr. Martha Rogers, also surpassed the prevailing dualistic view between health and disease in her conceptualization of unitary being. Her work asserts that being and becoming, spirit and matter, in fact all dualities, are artificial dichotomies. The Rogerian view of the world is as a single unitary energy field that generates, supports, and evolves. In her nonlinear world, things are defined as circular, cyclical, and rhythmical. She encouraged nurses to take their practice focus from procedural tasks and physical body symptoms to the higher realm of independent, health-promoting, noninvasive energy-based therapeutic systems. As part of the rhythmic world-process of higher frequency, the healer offers a compassionate, nonjudgmental, conscious presence that potentiates the field for a person's own self-healing (Rogers, 1970).

In each model, health, which encompasses both disease and nondisease, can be regarded as the explication of the underlying pattern of the person-environment. This shifting paradigm invites us to expand our viewpoint from looking at parts to looking at patterns. The pattern is information that depicts the whole, understanding the meaning of all the relationships at once. It is a fundamental attribute of the Universal Field, giving unity to the rich diversity within it (Capra, 1988, p. 17).

It is the pattern of our lives that identifies us, not the things that go into making up the pattern. Pattern is relatedness, which includes movement, diversity, and rhythm—energy waves of light and sound. This process is intimately involved in both energy exchange and change or transformation, for as energy is exchanged, the relationships within that pattern are altered (Young, 1976).

Within the past 40 years the acquisition of knowledge and information has accelerated at a pace beyond that seen upon this planet in all of recorded history. New information systems and the widespread access to books have given us an unprecedented accumulated wealth of knowledge. Through the process of triangulation, we can view a phenomenon of health through physical, psycho-social, and spiritual dimensions, giving an expanded view of reality.

Noted physician Larry Dossey has identified three eras that provide a framework for the medicine operational in the Western world today. The 1860s ushered in Era I, as science was incorporated into medical practice. During this period, the prevailing assumption was that health and illness were completely physical in nature, with a person's consciousness a by-product of the chemical, anatomic, and physiological aspects of the brain.

Era II emerged in the 1950s with therapies reflecting a growing awareness that a person's mind-consciousness, which includes thoughts, emotions, beliefs, attitudes, and meaning, exert an impact on the body. From this perspective, consciousness was viewed as a local phenomenon within the body, and in the present moment of a single lifetime.

Era III, the newest and most advanced, is nested within the quantum physics paradigm. Here consciousness is seen as nonlocal and not bound to one individual body. In this world the minds of humankind are spread throughout space and time. They are infinite, immortal, omnipresent, and ultimately, one. In this space a person is raised above the day-to-day level of control to experience a transpersonal experience outside of the local self (Dossey, 1982). As Dossey's rich research demonstrates, healing is affected by building bridges of consciousness with intercessory prayer, certain emotions (i.e., love, compassion), shamanic healing, and miracles. His observation is:

> We have nothing to lose by a reexamination of fundamental assumptions of our models of health; on the contrary, we face the extraordinary possibility of fashioning a system that emphasizes life instead of death, and unity and oneness instead of fragmentation, darkness and isolation. (Dossey, 1993, p. 86)

In this era, we are invited to become aware, each moment, of our inner and outer experiences, of our thoughts and assumptions, and of their impact on our world. The therapeutic potential of the mind becomes increasingly clear, fostering a knowing that all therapies and all people contain a transcendent quality that cultivates healing. In this space we cocreate and share the healing experience.

THE HUMAN BODY RE-ENVISIONED: AN INTEGRATED FIELD OF ENERGY

As our understanding of health and consciousness grows, we begin to see the human body and its relationship to the quantum world more clearly. Energy is wave and particle, light and sound. It begins as silence and formless form, slowly changing in composition as its vibratory rates are reduced. A new vision of light extends our understanding of the journey of inorganic and organic matter from subtle energy to a frozen form of light—matter. This then provides the foundations for this new medicine and a new psychology.

Since the beginning of time humanity has utilized the energy and power of the sun. The human body is a living photocell that is energized by the sun's light. Nobel Prize winner Szent-Gyorgyi recognized the power of light and color on the human body, concluding that "all of the energy taken into our bodies is derived from the sun" (Szent-Gyorgyi, 1968). Many enzymes and hormones involve the processing of light energy, causing dynamic reactions in the body. Light striking the body significantly alters basic biological cellular functioning and movement across cellular membranes. The energetic network, representing our physical/cellular framework, is organized and nourished by light.

At the cellular level, the wave patterns set in motion by light striking the body stimulate the integral membrane proteins embedded in the cell membrane. The two classes of IMP complexes include *receptor proteins* and *effector proteins*. The receptor proteins act as antennae that read vibrational energy fields such as light, sound, and wave frequencies. The receptor changes shape and function, depending on the vibration striking the body, carrying its message into the cell. At this point the effector proteins engage in the appropriate life-sustaining response. Thus the function of cells is derived from the movements of their "protein gears."

The interface between environmental signals and behavior-producing cytoplasmic proteins is the cell membrane, which acts as the cell's brain. Crystals, structures with molecules arranged in regular and repetitive fashion, transmit energy waves. Hard crystals are resilient minerals such as diamonds and rubies. Fluid crystals have molecules in a similar organized fashion and are found in digital watch faces and laptop computer screens. The cell membrane is a liquid crystal semiconductor with gates and channels, much like a computer chip. Both computers and cells are programmable, with the programmer outside of the computer/cell (Lipton, 2005, p. 90).

The protein complexes are the "perception switches" that stimulate the cell to respond in very basic ways to the potassium, calcium, oxygen, glucose, histamine, estrogen, toxins, light, or any number of other stimuli in their environment. When the cells respond, they release into the environment signals that influence the behavior of other cells within the ecosystem, creating a coordinated response. In living organisms, cells live in community, where they share their "awareness" and coordinate their behaviors by releasing signal molecules into the environment. All cells commit to a common plan of action that is coordinated by the brain, assuring survival of the host organism.

In her compelling work, *Molecules of Emotion,* Pert (1998) determined that the same neural receptors found in the brain were present on most of the body's cells. She demonstrated that the mind is not focused in the head, but is distributed via signal molecules throughout the entire body. Along with feedback from the body's environmental information, molecules of emotion can be generated by the brain, and can override the biological system. A self-conscious mind can bring health or disease to the body if excessive stress is generated; beliefs control biology.

Our perceptions, whether accurate or not, strongly impact our body-mind. The well known *placebo effect* has demonstrated that some people get well when they falsely believe they are getting medicine. While it is known that the mind, through positive suggestion, improves health, it is also clear that unconstructive suggestions can damage health. These negative effects are referred to as the *nocebo effect*. Studies have shown that some patients who understood they had a fatal diagnosis and were dying of cancer, were actually found—upon biopsy—to have very little disease present (Lipton, 2005, p. 142). By word and demeanor, physicians and other health care workers can convey hope-deflating messages to their patients. Positive and negative beliefs not only impact health, but every aspect of life. And over time our biology adapts to those beliefs.

All of these perspectives are demonstrating more about the functioning of the human brain and how internal neurological structures relate to the expression of human consciousness. Simultaneously, scientific visionaries like Pribram (1998) are uncovering new relationships between chemistry, physics, and human physiology, modeling how a simple chemical reaction can contribute to creation of new order in neurological organization through laser physics and holography.

The holographic model of the universe gives a new foundation for comprehending the unseen energy interconnections between all things. At a macroscopic level we are all constructed from the same subatomic building blocks. At a microcosmic level we are each complex, yet uniquely arranged aggregates of the same particularized energy field. Holography is shorthand for wave interference—the language of the Universal Field.

Einstein's theory guides us into this unfolding world of energy through the use of laser light. Incandescent light from a light bulb is diffuse and incoherent, spreading a soft light over a large area. Laser light is a very special type of coherent light that is extremely orderly, with all waves moving in step, like soldiers marching. When light is highly focused, it can burn a hole through steel.

A hologram is made by sending a single laser beam through an optical beam splitter, creating two laser beams from the original one. When the pure, unaffected laser beam meets the reflected light from the second one, through a process of mirrors and plates, an interference pattern is created. This interference pattern is produced by the waves of one beam mixing and interacting with the waves of the other beam. The interference pattern created by laser light and captured on photographic film is what forms the hologram. When a pure beam of laser light is shone on any part of the photographic film, a three-dimensional view of the entire object is seen. Thus, a hologram is an energy interference pattern where each piece of the picture contains the whole.

This pattern of interference is widely seen in nature. When two stones are dropped into a still pool of water, each creates a series of ever-expanding circular waves traveling outward. As the two groups of circular wave fronts meet, they interact and form an interference pattern. The pattern continues to expand, and at a specific point, the two merge into one larger, unified circle. Interference patterns can be constructive (energy-amplifying) when the waves are coordinated, as in harmonic resonance. Or the patterns can be destructive (energy-deflating), when the waves are out of sync.

The patterns of vibrational frequencies alter the physical and chemical properties of our body's structure. Talbot (1996) demonstrated that when we observe the world, the brain communicates with the rest of the body in the language of wave interference, the language of the spectrum domain—phase, amplitude, and frequency. In holographic fashion, the lens of the eye picks up certain interference patterns and converts them into three-dimensional images. We do not see the image on the back of our retina, but rather, we create and project a virtual three-dimensional image of the object out in space, in the same place as the actual object. In the act of observation we transform the timeless, spaceless world of interference patterns into the concrete and discrete world of space and time. At this point the image is collapsed and projected onto the retina, and our hand reaches out to touch the object where it really is, not inside our head.

After seeing, the brain processes the information in the shorthand of wave frequency patterns and, like a local area network, dispenses this information throughout the brain in a highly distributed system of connections where it is interpreted and stored. Storing the information in wave interference patterns is very efficient, allowing human memory to accommodate unimaginable quantities of data. It is projected that with wave interference patterns, the entire U.S. Library of Congress book collection, virtually every book ever published in English, would fit onto a large sugar cube.

The patterns of vibrational frequencies alter the physical and chemical properties of our body's structure (Endler, 1994). Memory is distributed throughout the brain, with numerous cells of the cerebral cortex tuned into certain frequencies. This makes pattern recognition possible. The brain also contains an "envelope," which limits the amount of wave information available to it as a protection against the limitless wave information contained in the Universal Field. When we are encouraged to push the envelope, it is a metaphor for enlarging the consciousness, or wave capacity of the brain.

As protons spin like magnets throughout the brain, they give off radiation. In this radiation is encoded wave information that can be used by the body to construct three-dimensional images of the body, the premise behind the MRI. Schempp's revolutionizing work showed that the imaging process worked with principles of holography, and acknowledged that this same principle was true for all biological systems. His unfolding work led to the notion of quantum holography.

Quantum fluctuations in the Universal Field hold infinite amounts of information, which can be recovered and reassembled into a three-dimensional image when perceived by a certain level of consciousness (Schempp, 1998). The common consciousness of humankind is much like an incandescent light, diffuse and incoherent. When one focuses with a high degree of intent, such as during meditation, laser thinking makes the information encoded in the universal energy field available to us all.

The holographic principle that every piece contains the whole is also seen in the cellular structure of all living beings. This model increases our understanding of the bioenergetic fields associated with the physical-chemical structure of the human body. Every cell contains the master DNA blueprint with enough information to create an entire human body, instructing each cell how to grow and function. This principle underlies the cloning of living cells (Gerber, 1995). What it does not do, however, is guide newly differentiated cells to their appropriate place in the developing embryo.

Epigenetics has uncovered a complex three-dimensional map of a bioenergetic field that surrounds the physical body. This field, or vital body, carries coded information for the spatial organization of the human body, as well as a roadmap for cellular repair (Pray, 2004; Silverman, 2004).

DNA blueprints passed on through genes are not set in concrete. Environmental influences such as nutrition, stress, and emotions can modify these genes, significantly altering their manifestation. In their compelling book on *The Lamarckian Dimension,* Jablonka and Lamb observed:

> In recent years, molecular biology has shown that the genome is far more fluid and responsive to the environment than previously supposed. It has also shown that information can be transmitted to descendants in ways other than through the base sequence of DNA. (Jablonka & Lamb, 1995, p. 178)

Multiple studies have demonstrated epigenetic mechanisms as a significant factor in a variety of diseases such as cancer and heart disease. One study showed that only 5% of cancer and cardiovascular patients can attribute their disorder to heredity (Willett, 2002). Malignancies are derived primarily from environmentally induced epigenetic alterations and not defective genes (Baylin, 1997; Jones, 2001; Kling, 2003; Seppa, 2000). The evidence increasingly shows a deep connection between an organism and its emotional environment.

Based on the continuing unfolding of science, contemporary physicians, such as Gerber, have envisioned a more comprehensive model for the human-energetic body. His model depicts the physical-vital-etheric interface between the organic-molecular form and the organizational energies of higher energy

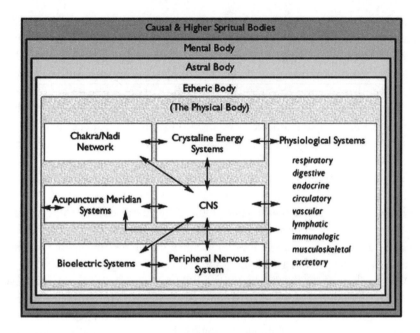

FIGURE 5.1   Human bioenergetic system.
SOURCE: Adapted from R. Gerber (1995), *Vibrational medicine: New choices for healing ourselves* (Santa Fe, NM: Bear and Company), p. 420.

sources. The total health of the human being is a product of a balanced and coordinated physical and higher-dimensional homeostatic regulatory system (Gerber, 1995). See Figure 5.1.

THE HUMAN MIND RE-ENVISIONED:
AN EXPANSIVE FIELD OF CONSCIOUSNESS

All living and inorganic things are shaped from the same matter that exists throughout the physical universe. Somehow consciousness participates in this entire process. We experience the physical world as external to us, while we also experience an inner world of awareness called soul consciousness. Consciousness itself is a form of energy, and at the highest levels it integrates all life processes. It is coextensive in the universe and exists in all matter. Each individual, and humankind as a species, are identified by their patterns of consciousness. A person does not *possess* consciousness, the person *is* consciousness. Consciousness is the ground of all being; the ground of both mind and matter (Newman, 1986).

Jantsch (1980, p. 40) defines consciousness as "the informational capacity of a system: the capacity of a system to interact with its environment." It is demonstrated by the degree of autonomy a system gains in dynamic relationship with its environment. Even the simplest autopoetic systems have a primitive form of consciousness. As the quality of consciousness increases, the number and variety of responses to the environment also expand. This is manifest as a greater repertoire of reactions with ease, speed, and grace. There is a greater refinement of response in terms of insight, context, and detail.

The mass consciousness of human awareness encompasses plant and animal ranges as well as astral and spiritual realms. The vibrational capacity of each level of being is not the same. Our reality depends on where we are on the spectrum of consciousness: level of consciousness determines reality. Increasing awareness creates a more intricate nervous system capable of environmental interaction in a more complex pattern. See Figure 5.2.

Viewing matter as a manifestation of consciousness reaffirms the unitary nature of body-mind, with mind representing faster high-frequency energy waves and body slower waves of lower amplitude. "Absolute Consciousness is a state in which contrasting concepts become reconciled and fused. Movement and rest fuse into one at the Source" (Bentov, 1978).

The new model for human-energy physiology includes consciousness at various stages of expression in each human being. Individual perception is uniquely different within each of the three spheres of consciousness: objective, subjective, and intermediary worlds. Our personal stage of development is described in terms that relate to our inner and outer perceptional capacity within those three spheres. Continuing spiritual development of the soul occurs as we increase the incorporation of higher levels of awareness into our basic human condition in the objective world of form (Fisher, 1996, vol. 1, pp. 58–62). See Figure 5.3.

- The Objective Universe: *Essence of Body,* the concrete world of form, is experienced as the body, personality, and mind-ego. It is the outer, objective manifestation of consciousness, whose energy levels are at sufficiently low orders of vibration to allow consciousness to experience and express itself in definite life-forms and life-experiences.
- The Subjective Universe: *Essence of Divine,* the abstract spiritual world of being, is experienced as our spiritual ego residing within our core self. It is the inner, subjective manifestation of consciousness, whose energy source is our causal body. Energy vibrations are so rapid that they are experienced as silence or formless form. Slowly

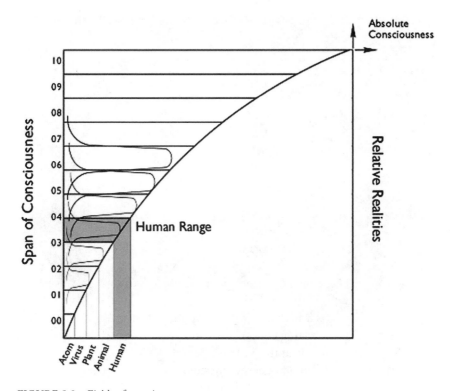

FIGURE 5.2   Fields of consciousness.
SOURCE: Adapted from I. Bentov (1978), *Stalking the wild pendulum* (New York: E. P. Dutton), p. 80.

they descend through seven planes of consciousness with increasingly slower wave patterns until physical manifestation is achieved.

- The Intermediate Sphere: *Essence of Mind,* the intermediate mental world of thought, is the medium for the impression of germinal thought forms from the higher abstract world into material manifestation in the concrete world. It functions as the focal point through which the soul contacts, controls, and dwells within the lower vehicle's form of the personality.

- The Soul: *Essence of Being,* our unique spark of life, is home of the divinity of each person. It serves as the coordinate in time and space of our causal body. Anchored in a sixth-dimensional space vortex outside the heart chakra, it is unseen by humans, who can perceive only four-dimensional forms (Prophet & Spadaro, 1995). The soul serves as the unifying force integrating human consciousness between its concrete physical and abstract spiritual experiences in this lifetime. When this coalescing force field is in effect, intuition—our inner

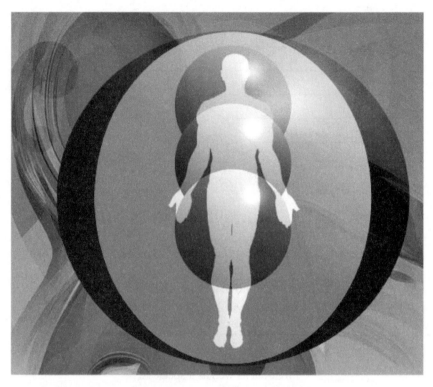

FIGURE 5.3   Spheres of consciousness.
SOURCE: Adapted from B.S. Fisher (1996), *Man, grand reflection of greater cosmos: Studies in occult anatomy.* (Vol.3) (Prescott, AZ: Subru Publications), p. 15.

wisdom—is awakened. This deeper knowing transcends the limitations of thought.

- The Causal Body: *Vehicle of Consciousness* is the outer sheath of our entire body-mind-spirit. Shaped like a luminous egg, it is the repository of the essence of all our previous life experiences. Home of our spiritual ego, which is a composite of all experiences across multiple lives, this vehicle is the interface through which our energetic vibratory patterns interact with the universe in a specific wave interference pattern that is our identity signature in the cosmos.

Spirit interacts with, and manifests through, the many forms of physical matter. The journey of spirit through the worlds of matter provides the strongest driving force for the evolutionary process.

It is the enriching endowing power of spirit that moves, inspires and breathes life into that vehicle we perceive as the physical body. A system of medicine which denies or ignores its existence will be incomplete, because it leaves out the most fundamental quality of human existence—the spiritual dimension. (Gerber, 1995, p. 419)

Realities of spirit do not negate laws of science, they only extend them to include higher-frequency dimensions, much as the incorporation of quantum principles into mechanical science increased the understanding and integration of various laws and principles that appeared disconnected in a three-dimensional world. The creative potential embedded within Absolute Consciousness (the Universal Zero-Point Field) has a self-organizing capacity that influences the being who perceives it.

The force of life continuously moves towards higher order, from planetary motion to the functioning of society. Prigogine's theory of dissipative structures (1976) demonstrates that while all dynamic systems fluctuate, rather than evening out, they eventually move to some supraordinate shift. The new order appears when a giant fluctuation is stabilized through an exchange of amplified energy with its environment. The functional and stable element is impacted by chance factors or critical events, coupled with an energetic surge, which results in a shift that produces physical mutations, behavioral or biological change.

Sheldrake (1981), a cellular biologist, demonstrated the mechanism for a shift in capacity for an individual as well as a species. His research showed that characteristic forms and behavior of physical, chemical, and biological systems are determined by invisible organizing fields acting across time and space. These morphogenetic fields are without mass or energy, and are cumulative in nature. Each generation can acquire learned tasks more easily than the last because of capacity embedded within this field. At some critical juncture, the acquired function is transcended into higher order and form because a morphogenetic field has been enlarged; this is the evolutionary nature of life.

These new models give us a view of the human body as a complex system composed of both matter and energy that is intertwined at multiple levels of reality. The image of the body as five nested hierarchies was discovered in India as part of the Vedanta literature. It also appears in Judaic tradition as part of the Kabala, as well as in the ancient mystery schools of Egypt (Bly, 1977; Frawlely, 1989; Svoboda & Lade, 1995). See Figure 5.4.

Human energy fields are composed of five nested levels of consciousness (Fisher, 1996; Goswami, 2004): gross physical, vital etheric, desire emotional, mental reflective, which houses archetypal patterns, and the causal body, which houses the spiritual ego. A level always occurs in groups of seven and can be divided into three upper and four lower groupings. Three lower levels are basic in nature, the fourth borderland is neutral, and three higher regions are chiefly expansive in nature.

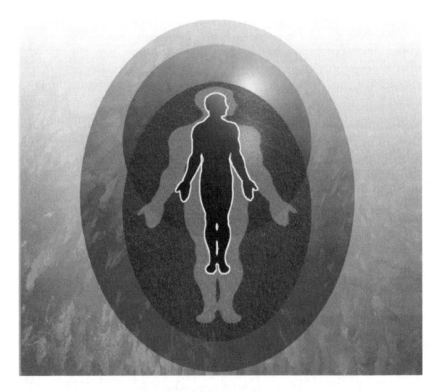

FIGURE 5.4   Human energy fields.

1. *The Gross Physical Body* is the coarsest level, an inert mineral machine, penetrated atom-for-atom by the vital body. It is the most organized and highly evolved, as well as the most highly crystallized of all matter forms in the universe. Each human body, the medium through which consciousness experiences life, is unique because of its physical structure. It serves as the receptor and transmitter through which are expressed the vital, emotional, and mental principles that originate in the subtle bodies that surround and inform it. It can be further developed through proper nutrition, rest, and exercise.

The physical level of disease occurs when the body's normal chemistry or physics goes awry. It also can be impacted by external agents such as microbes or trauma. Allopathic medicine, like classic physics, is very appropriate in treating mechanical and traumatic injuries, especially when immediate results are needed. Conventional medicine with its practices of surgery, drugs, and radiation assists with control of physical symptoms.

2. *The Vital Etheric Body,* an exact copy of the physical body, permeates through and follows the contours of the body while extending 3–5 centimeters beyond it. It is made from a colorless, volatile liquid, ether, often referred to

as the aura. Morphogenesis creates the vital body surrounding the physical body through access to nonphysical and nonlocal energy fields, whose main vortex is located near the spleen. This energy wrapper provides the structural and functional blueprints for the forms and programs of various organic structures, including the physical body. It guides the process of differentiation of a single-celled embryo into a biological body of discriminate organs. The blueprints are designed to guide vital body functions as well as maintenance, reproduction, and so on. Thus, organs are a representation of vital body blueprints of various morphogenetic fields (Fisher, 1996, vol. 1, pp. 2–4, 29–34; Mindell, 2004).

The three-dimensional vital body serves two purposes; it vitalizes the dense physical body, and it functions as an intermediate for the transmission of force-matter (coalescing energy that is turning into form) from the emotional and mental bodies to the physical brain and nervous system.

Current discussions in the scientific world are exploring the electromagnetic and gravitational force field of energy through the "string theory" paradigm (Green, 1999). It states that each quantum of energy is, in the final analysis, not a point, but rather a tiny, vibrating, one-dimensional loop similar to a very thin rubber band. Everything at the microscopic level consists of combinations of vibrating strands whose mass and force changes are determined by its vibratory pattern. Spirillae are the fundamental energy patterns through which various levels of energy (consciousness) are manifest throughout the universe. See Figure 5.5.

Emerging as a vital life force from the sun, energy spirillae are converted into the form of "vitality globules" as energy nourishment for the body (Fisher, pp. 23–25). These globules, etheric corpuscles, are absorbed by the vital body through force center openings (chakras) located just outside the physical body. The largest vortex is located near the spleen chakra. Just as a prism refracts light waves into seven colors representing the differing vibratory levels of light-energy, the spleen refracts particles (frozen light) into seven color globules of vital life force, which nourishes the seven chakra centers along with the specific endocrine glands and nerve structures they support. Simultaneously, excess vital life force and depleted etheric atoms, some chemical molecules, and microorganisms are eliminated through the vital aura, detoxifying the physical body, much as the circulatory system supports the physical body. Conservation and appropriate use of our vital force is essential to physical and extrasensory (emotional-mental) health. See Figure 5.6.

The vital body's second and higher function is the transmission of emotional/mental force-matter. It organizes and separates the higher ethers, concerned with sense perception and memory, from the lower ethers, involved with vitalizing,

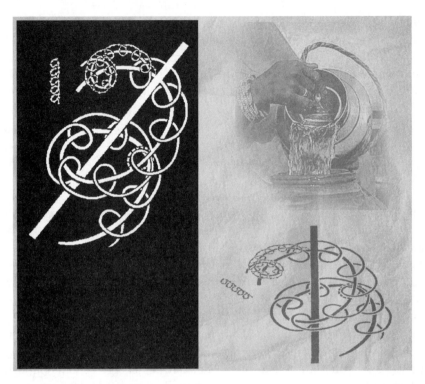

FIGURE 5.5   Energy spirilla.
SOURCE: Adapted from B.S. Fisher (1996), *Man, grand reflection of greater cosmos: Studies in occult anatomy* (Vol.3) (Prescott, AZ: Subru Publications), p. 21.

maintaining, and propagating the dense physical body. The lower part remains with the dense body to keep it alive, while the higher part is used by the ego as an organ of sense-perception, serving as the foundation of the body-mind. It can be strengthened through repetition of aesthetic and altruistic practices.

Each vital body is unique because of conditioning. Certain blueprints are used more than others, creating a pattern of personality. This etheric double serves as a medium for the life force, which affects vitality, assimilation and growth, excretion and detoxification, sense perception, and memory of immediate life events, our *body-mind* impressions.

Disease is a manifestation of disrupted body plans in the morphogenetic field, resulting in imbalances between physical and vital bodies. As this is the body sensation level of consciousness, illness elicits certain feelings or symptoms that accompany the recognizable physical components. Homeopathy, as well as Eastern Ayurveda and Chinese Medicine, are focused on treating the vital body. Restoring the blueprints takes more time than addressing physical

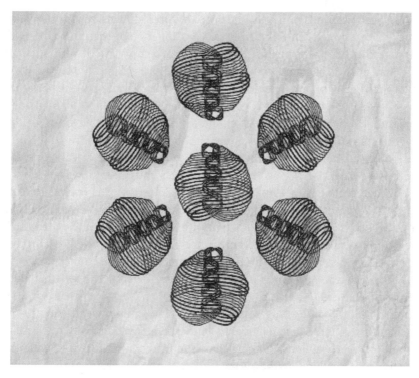

FIGURE 5.6   Vitality globules.
SOURCE: Adapted from B.S. Fisher (1996), *Man, grand reflection of greater cosmos: Studies in occult anatomy* (Vol. 3) (Prescott, AZ: Subru Publications), p. 25.

symptoms. Often a blending of conventional and holistic care in a compatible fashion begins to foster healing at the deeper levels of being.

3. *The Desire Emotional Body* serves as the medium for consciousness to experience and express desires, urges, emotions, and higher aspirations. This body extends 5–10 centimeters beyond the physical body and has a clearly defined boundary, its outer boundary being ovoid or egg-shaped. Serving as the seat of our volitional nature, its major function is to impel action. The emotional body contains forcefields roughly corresponding to those of the vital body, the main vortex being located near the liver.

The emotional body functions as our vehicle of feelings stimulated by coarse desires and wishes, or through emotions. The inside of this energy membrane is a field of constant motion, with differing clusters of coalescing energy (force-matter) flowing in a dance of joining and separation. As this body attracts thought forms, it crystallizes them into emotional structures, which influence the energy environment at the physical level of existence through receptor proteins.

The desire world is primarily one of color, a four-dimensional world where time, space, motion, and gravitational laws differ from the physical world. Here vision is four-dimensional, with objects being viewed from all sides simultaneously. The rapid circulation within the field precludes formation of localized centers of perception; emotions are free floating feelings as they are sensed all along the outer edge of the ovoid border of the emotional body. Here subtle attraction and repulsion, interest and disinterest are born.

Thoughts and emotions impact the vital body primarily through the central nervous system and the crown chakra. In an emotionally healthy person the flow of particle-wave exchange is effortless and light. However, a burst of negative emotions or aggression forms a clotting of this energy, causing stagnation from loss of flow, much as a stroke in the vascular system of the physical body. Negative mental activity impacts the body directly through the brain's connection to the central nervous system as well as through newly discovered psychoneuroimmunology neuropeptide connections.

The mind reacts to stress-producing agents, determining whether their effects will have an adverse reaction to the vital and physical body. An individual develops conditioned responses over time, ascribing meaning to the event with a patterned mental quality. The hyperactive mind will intellectualize and control emotions, burying the issue in the subconscious, while the sluggish mind will ignore the event, placing it into the realm of the subconscious through marginalization. A healthy balance of mind and emotion that transcends conditioning in a creative and fresh way is essential for healing at this level. Restoring balance at this level involves mind-body healing methods such as meditation, biofeedback, and yoga.

While the mind may be the originating cause of disease, body-mind healing through control of emotions, behaviors, and images will be inadequate when illness represents an imbalance at the higher level of the mental body.

4. *The Mental Reflective Body* is the third layer of the aura, reflecting the body of thought, knowledge, and experience. Extending 10–20 centimeters beyond the body around the head and shoulders, it flows from the top of the head downward in a yellow halo-form. The mental body is our vehicle of concrete thought, comprised of particles that are sensitive and responsive to the vibrations of thought forms emanating from the body-mind. It is the easiest to modify and purify quickly because of its low degree of organization and crystallization.

This is preeminently a world of tone; good music inspires us because it brings our awareness to our thought world, the *true home of the human mind*. It is a five-dimensional world, the added dimension being consciousness of more than one possibility within an event. It allows us to make more intelligent choices from the clear head in a difficult situation, versus the perspective of more limited four-dimensional consciousness in which only one possibility at a time can be seen in linear fashion.

Mind is the connecting point between the lower realm of concrete thought and the higher realm of abstract thought. It is here, in the organized and specialized body of the seven-layered thought world, that a bridge connects the four lower bodies (which comprise the personality-ego) with the causal body (spiritual ego). The lower aspect, the first three levels of the thought world, contain the concrete mind, with a sufficiently low vibratory rate to serve as a medium for impressions of thought and sensation. The higher aspect, the top three levels of the thought world, contains the abstract mind with an energy level of such high vibration that it cannot be molded into thought forms. It serves as a medium for germination of abstract ideas and broad concepts. The focal point, the intermediate fourth level, is the point of our focused awareness, shifting between the two spheres of the mental body, weaving inner and outer intelligence into a larger whole. See Figure 5.7.

The lower aspect of our mental body connects with our sense-organs, forming the *body-mind,* which responds to environmental entities (internal and external), which act on the body. We embody seven senses: sight, touch, hearing, smell, taste, the immunosystem, and the endocrine system. Body

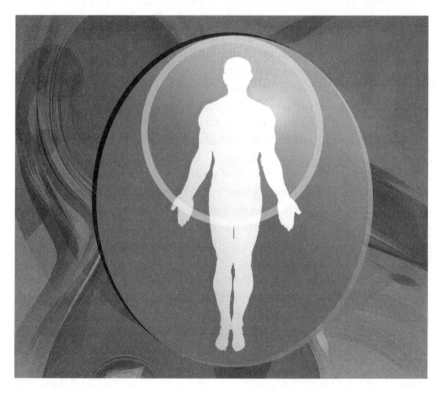

FIGURE 5.7   Mental reflective body.

awareness notifies the brain (physical brain or cell receptors) that something is in the environment. Externally we react (move hand from hot stove), while internally a toxic invader alerts the immunosystem or a stressful event compels the endocrine system to prepare the body for quick response. The concrete mind interprets the origin and significance of the event, deciding if the issue is threatening or enabling, guiding the body-mind in an appropriate reaction.

The higher aspect of our mental body is accessed through aesthetic or abstract thoughts, performing its most important function as the gateway through which the spiritual ego contacts, controls, and dwells within the four lower vehicles that form the personality.

5. *The Causal Body:* a theosophical term, this is viewed as the outer sheath, or vehicle of consciousness of the spiritual ego. Viewed as a blue oval extending 50–60 centimeters outside the physical body, it surrounds and embraces all bodies of consciousness. The causal body holds the archetypes for our uniqueness, forming our inner identity. It has a very resilient outer skin of protective film with an elastic capacity, which allows it to stretch and change without breaking. This serves as a protection against external forces and influences, while also providing the connection point to the universal energy field; the Source.

The causal body is the home of our threefold spiritual ego; love-wisdom, will-power, and active intelligence. This is a six-dimensional world with the addition of consciousness, which facilitates identifying all possibilities existing at once. This highest form of expression is our immortal one, the seat of our individuality, which persists from life to life, the vehicle of consciousness of the reincarnating soul. Intuition, referred to as inner wisdom, gives us access to the repository of all knowledge, faculties, and spiritually worthwhile experiences accumulated during many lifetimes.

Our spiritual ego grows in power, wisdom, and capacity by assimilating the essence of experience gained in successive lifetimes as soul qualities extracted from experience in the lower bodies of form, our personality. The distillation of the essence of our bodily experiences provides the energetic nourishment for our spiritual nature to acquire permanent patterns of vibration in the seed atoms of the causal body, as the basis for personal transformation. It also is the home of spiritual qualities such as peace and compassion, which are equally present in all human beings.

6. *Seed Atoms* are the relatively permanent energy forms that constitute our soul. They hold the universal archetypes, referenced by Plato and Jung (Jung, 1971; Plato, 1928), of our individual lives. See Figure 5.8.

Seed atoms are crystal forms of spiritual anatomy, which contain all attributes and knowledge acquired through all evolutions of the consciousness cycles. Emanating from their storehouse in the causal body, they are implanted in the fetus during quickening, between the 18th and 21st days

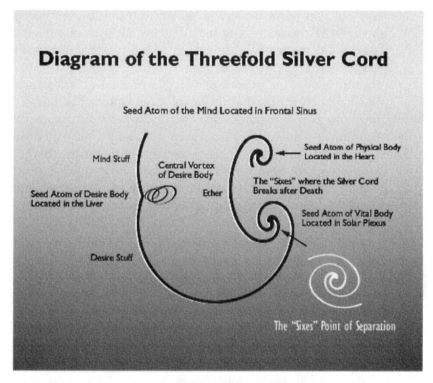

FIGURE 5.8   Seed atoms. Diagram of the threefold silver cord.
SOURCE: Adapted from B.S. Fisher (1996), *Man, grand reflection of greater cosmos: Studies in occult anatomy* (Vol.3) (Prescott, AZ: Subru Publications), p. 6.

of fetal development. Located at strategic points within the physical body, patterns of this life experience are impressed upon the seed atoms, similar to recording information on a hard drive in the computer (Fisher, 1996, vol. 3, pp. 5–8).

- The seed atom of the physical body is located in the left ventricle of the heart. Freshly aerated blood enters from the lungs, carrying holographic pictures of all life events, taken in through the air we breathe, carried by the blood, and ultimately recorded by the permanent physical seed atom in the heart. Those impressions we did not consciously note—that is, were not attentive to—constitute the unconscious mind.
- The seed atom of the vital body is located in the solar plexus, by the spleen, capturing all modifications made to the vital blueprint throughout the life span.

- The seed atom of the desire body is located in the central vortex of the desire/emotional body in the vicinity of the liver, recording all emotional thoughts and urges as well as higher aspirations experienced in our lived experience.
- The seed atom of the concrete mind is located in the frontal sinus, in the energy field surrounding the pineal gland, capturing all thoughts, ideas, and creative ventures crafted within the current life-journey.
- The silver cord is the energy connection that joins the four seed atoms of the personality. Entering our body through the crown chakra, it flows through the central nervous system to the heart chakra. It serves as the connecting link between all of our bodies of consciousness, remaining attached to the physical body throughout this lifetime.

The transfer of life experiences occurs upon experiencing death, starting with the rupture of the seed atom of the heart. Recent life impressions stored in subconscious memory are transferred as *soul qualities* to the vital body seed atom in the solar plexus, much as we make a copy of a CD recording. The personality ego then perceives an unemotional panoramic review in reverse order, of the life ended from all stored seed atoms. This process takes approximately 3 days.

Rupture of the silver cord occurs upon completion of the transfer and life review. The ego becomes separated from the physical and etheric bodies and the supply of the vital life force is cut off, causing both bodies to disintegrate. The spiritual ego now moves in stages through the remaining energy bodies until it comes to rest in the causal body, with all the information and inspiration of the life encoded into the soul.

During this life experience, spiritual distress can be the originating point for physical illness. Patterns encoded in the personality and spiritual ego include both assets and shortcomings of all previous lifetimes as well as the current one. Correction of our imbalances is the goal of personal transformation as we grow in capacity during our lifetime. True spiritual healing involves integration, the recovery of a sense of wholeness through the reconnection of the personality and the spirit. Integration of ego-separateness eliminates vital body imbalances due to emotional preferences, restoring balance to all bodies of consciousness. This process of enlightenment is referred to in esoteric healing traditions as spiritual alchemy (Hall, 2003).

The causal body serves as the spiritual boundary that allows us to meld and become one with the Source. Spirit is a seven-dimensional consciousness where we realize possibilities beyond those of our soul experience. In this state we create our own reality.

7. *The Chakra System: Prana*, the vital life force, is a form of the universal energy field that originates from the sun. It is transformed into vitality globules,

which serve the same purpose in the etheric vital body as red blood corpuscles serve in distributing oxygen to the cells of the physical body.

We are capable of feelings of great vitality and aliveness, or deep fatigue and low energy. The activation of the vital blueprint is sensed as an energy movement we experience as sensory feelings within the physical body. This vitality can most easily be detected at certain points in the body; the chakra points. These chakra points are located close to a major nerve plexus and a major endocrine gland. Serving as an energy transformer, they step down energy of one frequency to a lower level, which can be transported by specific subtle energetic channels into the cellular structure of the physical body. It is at these points where vital energy is made into physical representations (Motoyama, 1981). See Figure 5.9.

The major chakras are situated in a vertical line ascending from the base of the spine to the head.

- The lowest, called the *root chakra*, creates the necessary foundation for life and living. Activated at birth when the umbilical cord is cut,

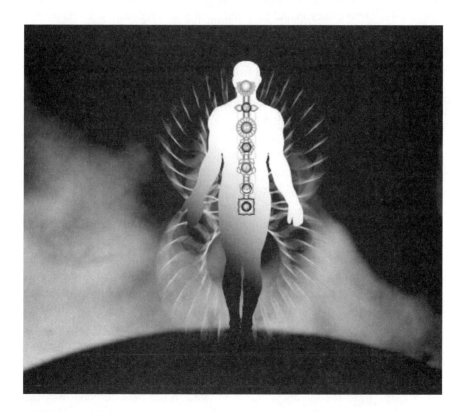

FIGURE 5.9   Chakras.

the vital energy channeled into this chakra creates a deep connection with the world and the sacral-coccygeal nerve plexus. Located at the base of the tailbone (red in color), it energizes the physical body and lower extremities, including the feet, to establish and maintain physical connection with the world.

- The second, the *sacral chakra,* activates all senses, providing sexual and creative energy as well as instinctual and emotional feelings. It boosts our awareness and desire for beauty, relationships, and pleasure, establishing a healthy enthusiasm for being alive. Located in the lower abdomen (orange in color) near the spleen, it energizes the reproductive organs, bladder, and lower intestines as well as sacral nerve plexus, while also expressing the *eros* aspect of love.

- The third, or *solar plexus chakra,* lies in the upper abdomen below the tip of the sternum. This connection serves as a gateway for emotions and the projection of volitional energy such as anger. Intellectually it determines our level of decision making, direction, and personal power while emotionally it guides our ability to trust our most fundamental intuition and instincts. Our self-image and personality are formed by the masks, characteristics, and attitudes we adopt to navigate through the world, providing the determination, conviction, and courage to achieve the life we are seeking. Located close to the naval (yellow in color), it energizes the spleen, adrenals, pancreas, stomach, upper intestines, gallbladder, liver, and lower back as well as the solar plexus nerve center.

- The fourth, or *heart chakra,* is found in the midsternal region directly over the heart and thymus gland. This chakra is the point of transformation, the center of balance. It connects the lower body-mind with higher soul-wisdom. It serves as the center for balance for the entire physical-vital-mental system, fostering altruism, compassion, forgiveness, understanding, generosity, empathy, caring, and love. Here we open our heart to connect with others, feeling joy and unity. It stimulates our highest ideals and desires for others and the world. When balanced, we are able to open up, partake of, and share with the universe. Located at the center of chest (rose pink in color), it energizes the thymus, heart, circulatory system, breast, and blood flow as well as the heart plexus nerve center. It, along with the solar plexus and crown chakras, are the only three that receive psychic and spiritual energies directly from higher dimensions. It expresses the *philos* aspect of love.

- The fifth, the *throat chakra,* is situated in the neck directly over the Adam's apple, covering the thyroid gland and larynx. This serves as the center of expression and aesthetic creativity, as well as our ability to connect with the creative expression of others—which lays the foundation for understanding. It is the center for negotiation, discussion, teaching, and learning. It is also the gateway to the world, moving us from our subjective perspective to other points of view. Expression is an agent for progress, evolution, peace, and healing relationships. Located at the back of neck (blue in color), it energizes the thyroid, parathyroid, and hypothalamus, throat, neck, trachea, esophagus, mouth, teeth, and ears as well as the cervical ganglia medulla nerve plexus.

- The sixth, the *brow chakra,* is located in the mid-forehead slightly above the bridge of the nose. This center enhances quality of thought and all aspects of mind, including intuitive wisdom. It focuses our ability to see accurately in life, to analyze, think, reason, perceive, understand, discern, dream, imagine, and visualize. It is the center of personal vision, fostering focused clarity without distortion. Located at the third eye between the eyebrows (green in color), it energizes the pituitary gland, head, eyes, and all sense organs as well as the autonomic nervous system. This center embodies the root essence of the first five chakras and expresses the *agape* aspect of love.

- The seventh, the *crown chakra,* is located on top of the head, serving as the center for our highest spiritual consciousness and personal expression, connecting us to the Source of life. It opens the way for us to become a bearer of light in the world, focusing our attention on the spiritual meaning of life. Such a perspective begins to erase the imagined demarcation between what is spiritual and what is not. Located at the top of head (gold in color), it energizes the pineal gland, brain stem, spinal cord, and central nervous system. Representing inner wisdom, it combines with the brow and higher octave of the throat chakra, creating the spiritual triangle through which the three higher aspects of consciousness (wisdom, will, and activity) are expressed.

These primary chakras begin as centers within the vital body. They are connected to each other and to portions of the physical-cellular structure through fine threads of subtle energy called *nadis.* These nadis represent an extensive network of fluid-like energies that parallel bodily nerves in their abundance and function. Various sources report up to 72,000 nadis or etheric channels of energy in the subtle anatomy of human beings. Interwoven with the physical nervous system, they affect the nature and quality of nerve transmission through the brain network. Dysfunction of the chakra system impacts the quality of the nervous system, as well as the attached endocrine gland and nerve plexus necessary for optimal human functioning (Montoyama, 1981, pp. 93–98).

Wellness is a multidimensional phenomenon requiring homeostasis within the concrete physical body as well as the functioning of the mapped blueprints of the vital body. It also requires a continuous flow of vital energy movement into the physical body with a balancing of various aspects of this *prana* energy. When a dynamic state of balance and harmony exist between the physical and energy aspects of our being, optimal well-being and vitality are experienced.

BALANCE: THE KEY TO VIBRANT WELL-BEING

Contemporary nursing practice requires two distinct functions: the clinical practice of the profession, and the modeling of what we seek for others in our own life. How healthy are you? What level of vitality and well-being is present in your current life situation? What balance is present in your life? What healing practices do you ascribe to in routines of your day?

All living systems move towards a state of stability and harmony with other systems. Because we consistently grow and change, we are in constant interchange with our environment in a disruptive way, moving in and out of balance in the perpetual dance of life. A sense of right timing and proper alignment infuses our connections and relationships with grace, filling our lives with a rhythm and harmony that is the hallmark of health.

The quantum science-based law of polarity states that from molecular to cosmic phenomena, all things exist as opposite electromagnetic fields, with a third neutral force in the center that is not accessible to direct observation or understanding. Nothing can exist except in relation to its opposite. The positive is forever transforming into the negative, while the negative is transforming into the positive; each power needs the other to exist. When things change, they move through a small neutral portal at the center. The emergence of new order, suggested by chaos theory, flows through this opening. When creating or managing health or change, pushing or pulling is a signal that alignment is not yet perfected. The act of honoring intuition that senses right timing is an essential capacity for living in balance (Koerner, 2004a, pp. 93–98).

Balance is a multifaceted diamond when viewed through the eyes of our diverse and beautiful world. A typical Western view of balance asserts that it is attained when there is physical, mental, and emotional harmony. A strong focus on physical and mental aspects of health helps us master the management of the material world, both our body and our life space.

Indigenous plains people focus on the emotional and spiritual dimensions of balance with their emphasis on thoughts, feelings, and the manifestation of expectations. All of these things arise from deeply held beliefs and attitudes. Finding the meaning embedded within a life event is the balancing force that guides and heals.

Lakota spiritual healer, Wanigi Waci, observed that polar opposites are the same thing in extreme, with each serving a valid function.

> We are spiritual beings who come to the material world for concrete experience. We come to experience the whole spectrum of emotions: joy and sorrow, pain and pleasure, love and betrayal. It is only by experiencing the opposites that our understanding of the phenomenon becomes whole and balanced. Each duality is the same element in differing degrees, so the key to learning resides in the ability to embrace each one fully. While the joy of friendship is meaningful, so is the sadness of tragedy. Cherish them equally and do not seek out one more than the other. When you can touch both poles with equivalent ease, you are living in harmony and balance, and the true lessons to be learned will be yours. (quoted in Koerner, 2004a, pp. 121–122)

Balance is found when you can stand in the middle in any circumstance, with no attachment or judgment, moving freely and adaptively across the continuum.

Chinese philosophy utilizes the yin-yang diagram to depict balance. It suggests that the universe is run by a single principle, the Tao or Great Ultimate. This principle divides into two forces that oppose one another in their actions: yin and yang. Together they accomplish change, which emerges through the most powerful point, the yo. Intersecting between yin and yang, the yo is the refining dimension that connects these two opposing forces. This flexible space creates a *dynamic balance* rather than balance in the static leveling-out sense. Living in the flow (yo) is the optimal state of balance, achieved by moving within the dynamic center of life rather than at a single polar point (Lao-Tzu, 1992).

In his compelling book, *No Boundaries,* Ken Wilbur compares a dynamic boundary to the sea. The ever-changing point of connection between land and ocean moves with the tide. He suggests that, rather than viewing a boundary as a line that keeps things in or out, the boundary can be seen as the point of connection. As we become more skilled at the subtle and immaterial realms, we can keep moving and managing the changing energy shifts in purposeful and meaningful ways (Wilber, 1985).

Exploration into the physical and spiritual domains of science and consciousness leave the nurse healer of contemporary twenty-first-century medicine with a wide array of tools and technologies to help foster a healing experience. Models for establishing and maintaining optimal health abound that can guide nurses in their own healing practices. From a centered and holistic perspective, they can then offer guidance and support to others on their own healing journey. Further, the blending of allopathic and integrative medicine with ancient spiritual wisdom and modern faith will offer a healing model to address all levels of body/consciousness in culturally sensitive ways, transforming the health of society and the earth.

From the cowardice that shrinks from new truth,
From the laziness that is content with half-truths,
From the arrogance that thinks it knows all truth,
O God of Truth, deliver us.

An ancient scholar

BIBLIOGRAPHY

Baylin, S. B. (1997). DNA methylation; Tying it all together: Epigenetics, genetics, cell cycle, and cancer. *Science, 277*(54), 1948–1957.

Bentov, I. (1978). *Stalking the wild pendulum.* New York: E. P. Dutton.

Bly, R. (1977). *The Kabir book.* Boston: Beacon.

Bohm, D. (1980). *Wholeness and the implicate order.* London: Routledge and Kegan Paul.

Capra, F. (1988). *The Tao of physics.* New York: Bantam.

Dossey, L. (1982). *Space, time and medicine.* Boulder, CO: Shambhala.

Dossey, L. (1993). *Healing words: The power of prayer and the practice of medicine.* San Francisco: HarperSanFrancisco.

Endler, P. C., et al. (1994). Transmission of hormone information by non-molecular means. *FASEB Journal, 8,* 400.

Fisher, B. S. (1996). *Man, grand reflection of the greater cosmos: Studies in occult anatomy.* (Vols. 1 and 3). Prescott, AZ: Subru.

Frawley, D. (1989). *Ayurvedic healing.* Salt Lake City, UT: Passage Press.

Gerber, R. (1995). *Vibrational medicine: New choices for healing ourselves.* Santa Fe, NM: Bear and Company.

Goswami, A. (2004). *The quantum doctor: A physicist's guide to health and healing.* Charlottesville, VA: Hampton Roads.

Green, B. (1999). *The elegant universe: Superstrings, hidden dimensions, and the quest for the ultimate theory.* New York: Vintage.

Hall, M. P. (2003). *The secret teachings of all ages: An encyclopedic outline of Masonic, hermetic, Qabbalistic, and Rosicrucian symbolical philosophy.* New York: Jeremy P. Tarcher/Penguin.

Jablonka, E., & Lamb, M. (1995). *Epigenetic inheritance and evolution: The Lamarckian dimension.* Oxford: Oxford University Press.

Jantsch, E. (1980). *The self-organizing universe.* New York: Pergamon.

Jones, P. A. (2001). Death and methylation. *Nature, 409,* 141–144.

Jung, C. G. (1971). *The portable Jung* (J. Campbell, Ed.). New York: Viking.

Kling, J. (2003). Put the blame on methylation. *The Scientist, 4,* 117–120.

Koerner, J. (2004a). Balance: compassionate engagement in society. *Nurse Leader, 4*(1), 28–31.

Koerner, J. (2004b). *Mother heal myself: An intergenerational healing journey between two worlds.* Santa Rosa, CA: Crestport.

Lao-Tzu. (1992). *Tao Te Ching: A new English version* (S. Mitchell, Trans.). San Francisco: HarperCollins.

Lipton, B. (2005). *The biology of belief: Unleashing the power of consciousness, matter, and miracles.* Santa Rosa, CA: Mountain of Love/Elite Books.

Mindell, A. (2004). *The quantum mind and healing.* Charlottesville, VA: Hampton Roads.

Montoyama, H. (1981). *Theories of the chakras.* Wheaton, IL: Theosophical Publishing House.

Newman, M. (1986). *Health as expanding consciousness.* St. Louis, MO: C. V. Mosby.

Pert, C. (1998). *Molecules of emotion: Why you feel the way you feel.* London: Simon and Schuster.

Plato. (1928). *Symposium* (A. Niehamas & P. Woodruff, Trans.). Oxford: Oxford University Press.

Pray, L. A. (2004). Epigenetics: Genome, meet your environment. *The Scientist,* 14–20.

Pribham, K. (1998). Autobiography in anecdote: The founding of experimental neuropsychology. In R. Bilder (Ed.), *The history of neuroscience in autobiography* (pp. 306–349). San Diego, CA: Academy Press.

Prigogine, I. (1976). Order through fluctuation: Self-organization and social system. In E. J. Jantsch & C. H. Waddington (Eds.), *Evolution and consciousness* (pp. 93–133). Reading, MA: Addison-Wesley.

Prophet, E. C., & Spadaro, P. R. (1995). *Your seven energy centers: A holistic approach to physical, emotional and spiritual vitality.* Corwin Springs, MT: Summit University Press.

Rogers, M. E. (1970). *An introduction to the theoretical basis of nursing.* Philadelphia: F. A. Davis.

Schempp, W. J. (1998). *Magnetic resonance imaging: Mathematic foundations and applications.* London: Wiley-Liss.

Seppa, N. (2000). Silencing the BRCA1 gene spells trouble. *Science News, 17,* 247.

Sheldrake, R. (1981). *A new science of life.* Los Angeles: Tarcher.

Silverman, P. H. (2004). Rethinking genetic determinism: With only 30,000 genes, what is it that makes humans human? *The Scientist,* 32–33.

Svoboda, R., & Lade, A. (1995). *Tao and Dharma: A comparison of Ayurveda and Chinese medicine.* Twin Lakes, WI: Lotus Press.

Szent-Gyorgyi, A. (1968). *Bioelectronics.* New York: Academic Press.

Talbot, M. (1996). *The holographic universe.* London: Harper Collins.

Wilbur, K. (1985). *No boundary: Eastern and Western approaches to personal growth.* Boston: Shambhala.

Willett, W. C. (2002). Balancing life-style and genomics research for disease prevention. *Science, 296,* 695–698.

Young, A. M. (1976). *The reflexive universe: Evolution of consciousness.* San Francisco: Robert Briggs.

CHAPTER 6

Quantum Healing

The Path of Integration

Perhaps each of us has a starved place,
each of us knows deep down what we need to fill that place.
To find the courage to trust and honor the search,
to follow the voice that tells us what we need to do,
even when it doesn't seem to make sense, is a worthy pursuit.

Sue Bender

Illness is part of the human health experience; no one gets through life without some form of physical ailment. Whether it's the common cold, a lingering chronic illness, or a life-threatening event, every living organism will inevitably encounter a moment when the body is suffering and in need of attention.

What have been your personal experiences with illness? An instructive paradox exists within our profession; at times we are the nurse and other times the person who is ill. Whether it is our self personally, or a family member or loved one, we each encounter illness at some point in our lives. It is important to reflect on the lessons learned and attitudes assumed, for, just like those we serve, we come to the healing experience with a set of beliefs and expectations that color the exchange in interesting ways.

Rites of passage form an integral part of many cultures worldwide, assisting and supporting their members through predictable stages of maturation. Rituals acknowledge important life changes such as birth, puberty, marriage, illness, and death; the rich markings of a person deeply engaged in living their journey. Unfortunately, Western society has displaced many traditions with the demands and expectations of day-to-day life in contemporary society. However, when the world stops, as it does when one is faced with a serious health crisis, their absence is palpable. Intuitively, at that juncture, we begin to create rituals around our own health and illness, a process designed to infuse meaning into our suffering.

Traditional allopathic methods of healing treat the immediate situation with interventions that manage the symptoms, without eradicating the root cause of suffering. As we come to understand the beautiful and dynamic body as a quantum entity, a nested hierarchy of varying levels of energy and consciousness, a new way of engaging with illness emerges. In this world we do not have to delve into the past to unearth the origins of our neurosis or traumas. We do not have to resort to distraction as an escape by filling our lives with endless activities or cultivate a positive mental attitude to drive out undesirable elements in our behavior. There is nothing to acquire; we have all we need within.

In this rich multidimensional world, which is our home, we can choose to treat the whole person, which includes the physical, emotional, mental, and spiritual aspects of our life, by inviting in the power of soul. The essence of soul consciousness influences the brain via the mind and touches all aspects of the person's nature. In this approach to healing, we invite symptoms and suffering into our space as our guide. We sit with sadness as it slowly offers the rich information that was ignored or suppressed for so long. We work with energy going into and out of the physical body as it navigates through the various levels of energy consciousness. And we recover the authentic qualities of the soul that were our birthright, fostering integration at the deepest levels. In short, we become whole.

THE HEALING PROCESS: RE-ESTABLISHING FLOW

The feeling of wonder begins with our own body. The closest that nature, others, and existence itself comes to us is through our own miraculous body. This material form holds the water of oceans, the fire of sun and stars, the air; our body is a gift from the earth (Osho, 2003). Mind is the inner unseen part of the body, while the body is an external manifestation of the mind; the body is the portal of the mind. The conscious mind comprises only 10% of our reality, while deeper truth is experienced in the loving communion between body and mind. When we relax into the flow of life, we are guided by the gentle and subtle promptings of our inner wisdom (the 90% of consciousness that lies below the level of normal awareness). Respect and harmony between body and mind manifest as vibrant health and vitality.

However, we are not the body; we are a conscious awareness that takes up residence in this concrete material form. We are a resident in the body temple, a communal gathering place created from the blending of earth (our body) and sky (our consciousness). When we have a healthy relationship to ourselves, as a witness-observer to our body-mind, we are aware of its needs and honor them. We are conscious of the language we use in speaking to and about our body. By honoring its needs and promptings we develop a deep trust in our inner wisdom, and a right alignment with the energetic flow of life occurs. If we ignore or marginalize symptoms, they will intensify as the body honors our focus, often at its own peril.

All disease is a result of disharmony between the body (form) and the vital life force (energy). The root cause of all illness is the inhibition of the flow of this force from the universal field, the Source. Most of the blockage occurs in the vital-etheric body and the desire-emotional body, with a lesser amount of illness coming from the mental-reflective body. True healing occurs when the obstruction to the energy flow is removed. Many physical body problems are the result of over-stressing this mechanism by forcing it to respond to the more subtle and subjective vibrations of our emotional world. This is where the mass consciousness of the majority of present humanity resides. Some physical conditions emerge from the disharmony acquired in connecting with the collective psyche of humankind.

Diseases emanating from the desire-emotional body primarily affect the autoimmune system and the central nervous system. Those rooted in the vital-etheric body manifest as congestion and misalignment of the nadis, the energy circulatory pathways in the etheric web. This results in either depletion of energy or over-stimulation, both of which cause disease and death. Those arising from the mental-reflective body emerge from erroneous or negative thinking, generating destructive thought-forms. These forms act directly on the desire-emotional body, which crystallizes negative emotions, producing one of the most potent causes of bodily enervation (Fisher, 1996, pp. 75–78).

Current diagnostic techniques focus on assessment and evaluation of the physical body. However, a comprehensive assessment of illness must include several dimensions beyond the physical symptoms if true healing is to be fostered. Evaluating the primary nature of the cause would include a consideration of factors that are psychic or subjective, inherited or genetic, as well as disharmonious with the human collective psyche. Methods of treatment expand beyond conventional allopathic medicine. While it remains a viable and often essential treatment form, others are also considered.

Infusion or redirection of vital energies is enhanced through Ayurveda practices developed in India, acupuncture and Chinese medicine, chakra balancing with homeopathy, and psychology. Mind-body medicine addresses issues around emotional and mental imbalance. Hypnosis, biofeedback, guided imagery, psychoanalysis, meditation, yoga, Christian Science and faith healing, all assist with slowing down the mind to reconsider the false meaning attributed to an event or issue, as well as facilitating management of stress (Goswami, 2004).

Quantum healing, the most profound and far-reaching form of healing, requires one fundamental action, to take a discontinuous quantum leap in our belief system. The mental belief we attach to something has a strong influence on its impact to our health (as in the placebo affect). Physical illness caused by mental meanings that impose disharmony on our vital and physical bodies requires a change in the meaning-context that the mind establishes for the malfunctioning to occur. The context for mental thinking comes from the consciousness of our mental-reflective body. Physicians Larry Dossey and Deepak Chopra, among others, have identified that self-healing at this level involves a quantum leap in consciousness:

> Many cures that share mysterious origins—faith healing, spontaneous remissions, and the effective use of placebo, or "dummy drugs"—also point toward a quantum leap. Why? Because in all of these instances, the faculty of inner awareness seems to have promoted a drastic jump—a quantum leap—in the healing mechanism. This is mediated by Higher Consciousness of the Spiritual Ego. (Chopra, 1989, p. 86)

This quantum leap is a creative act, coming from the highest level of our consciousness. It is the consciousness of the causal body, which has the requisite wisdom (encoded in our spiritual ego), the mechanism (choosing a new context in which to process the meaning of emotions), the power to discover what is needed (the ability to make a quantum leap of insight), and the power to manifest the insight by unlocking the blocked vital energy at the appropriate chakra, and thus, the physical organ. Our true healing capacity is a program of ultimate creativity, going through all the stages of the creative process, which ends in a change in the context of our life.

To foster such a shift, we might encourage the patient to research his or her own disease, with the assistance of a health care provider. The person would be invited to meditate upon it. Root causes of mental stress include the sense of deep urgency, rush, and hurry, coupled with anxiety and the pursuit of desires for accomplishment. A mind that is slowed down is more open and receptive, the first step towards creativity. Next, the person would begin to experiment with various mind-body medicine techniques, utilizing unlearned stimuli to generate uncollapsed possibility waves as unconscious processing occurs. Sooner or later a seemingly inconsequential trigger precipitates the quantum leap of insight: a corrective contextual shift in how the mind handles emotion occurs.

Freed from the restraints of mentalization and intellectualism, feelings and vital blueprints become functional once again, leading to sometimes dramatic healing of the illness. From a creative insight we are able to choose the healing path out of a myriad of possibilities generated by the unconscious processing. This choosing is the result of guidance from our inner wisdom, the integrative work of a unitive consciousness in the quantum self.

THE HEALING PATH: STAGES OF INTEGRATION

The curing model prevalent in contemporary society can be very beneficial. It offers us comfort in the form of symptom management, and time in which to do the more complex work of deeper healing. However, oftentimes it can deny rather than facilitate the possibility of healing. The processes used in curing are an attempt to control our experiences, moving them in a prescribed manner and direction towards a predetermined outcome. This process interferes with our ability to move into unsolicited experiences, the ones required for the restructuring of our lives. When this occurs, instead of experiencing the illness event as a step forward towards wholeness, its opposite occurs. However, when used as a stepping stone to multi-layered healing, curing can be very constructive.

Healing has little to do with removal of symptoms. Rather, it is an intimate and integrative process that encompasses the entire spectrum of our existence. This daunting journey requires the harmonious alignment of the physical, emotional, mental, and spiritual aspects of our being and how we relate to the world. The outcome of this integration is a greater sense of wholeness and vitality, wellness and soundness; the birthright of every living being (Schoch, 2005).

As quantum physics has demonstrated, a disruptive event offers the space for new order (Prigogine, 1976). Healing can be viewed as a process of rebuilding one's life anew from chaos and disorder. Psychiatrist Bendit observed:

> Healing is basically the result of putting right our wrong relation to our body, to other people....and to our own complicated minds, with their emotions and instincts at war with one another and not properly understood and accepted by what we call "I" or "me." The process is one of reorganization, reintegration of things which have come apart. (Bendit, 1973, p. 71)

The beginning of the healing journey finds us coming apart at the seams. As we begin to wake up and realize aspects of ourselves we could not previously acknowledge, a deep sadness sets in. By courageously continuing the journey deep into the territory called the self, we being to acknowledge our true condition. True intent to embark on the task of alignment gives our entire being permission to change. In a very natural and automatic way we initiate the release of old and worn-out thought patterns, we free blocked emotions and rigid ways of being. We develop a new sense of respect for who we really are, the essence of our latent capacities and the rhythms that are truly ours. Just as a flower opens in the spring, we quietly and naturally unfold and return to our authentic self. Nothing is taken out, nothing is added; we are already whole.

This daunting journey into healing moves through predictable stages, leaving in its wake a deep sense of fulfillment, accomplishment, and empowerment (Epstein, 1994). The journey is focused on our uniqueness. It involves surrender to both the inner and outer experiences that form our life. It promotes wholeness, which allows the natural rhythms and cycles of our life to be reinstated. It requires forgiveness of others, and offers forgiveness to our self.

Stage I: Embracing Our Suffering

Experienced as a different quality than pain, suffering marks the awareness that something is wrong. Pain is an awareness of discomfort manifest in symptoms of some fashion. Suffering, however, involves the sense of alienation from our true self, that something is wrong deep in our lives. Due to cultural and familial rules and messages, each of us has isolated certain aspects of ourselves, such as personality traits or painful childhood memories, from the rest of our body-mind. Often activated by a painful experience, the pattern for armoring and withdrawing inside of ourselves emerges as we prepare to bear something from which there is no escape.

In this stage we are not yet conscious enough to recognize the subtle but profound distinction between our sense of self and our suffering. The pain and discomfort of the moment narrows perspective; a three-dimensional space offers few options for reaction aside from conditioned patterns of response. Here memories of the past freeze our sense of self into a rigid and fixed entity that has been learned in painful events buried in our subconscious history.

Suffering is a natural by-product of a distorted sense of self. Our level of suffering is related to how we perceive the events in our lives. In this stage we lose touch with normal time-space perception. Time stands still. "Get the doctor." and "What took you so long?" are common comments heard. There is an intensified fear of the future. "What is going to happen to me now?" or, "Will this happen again?" are frequent remarks. This stage is very enveloped in the mind, a totally self-focused state of consciousness. There is a felt interference pattern in the connection with the core self and the way one is living. In essence, an inner voice is crying, "Wake up!" warning us that something is wrong.

Initially we resist suffering through denial, escape, intellectualizing, or distracting ourselves from direct experience. The turning point is the simple act of surrender. Growing weary of the struggle, we ultimately stop fighting and begin to work with the suffering. Here a critical shift in consciousness takes place. Roberts has observed:

> Here begins the cauterizing, the burning through to the deepest center of being, which is painful and shattering to all aspects of self. The deep deterministic reins of self-control have been taken away and the willpower that glued together this fragile unity has dissolved. From here on, the reins of our destiny are in the hands of a greater power.... With no place else to go, nowhere else to turn, we have no choice. (Roberts, 1985, p. 43)

This is an internal spiritual or mental emergency that cannot effectively be treated or cured. Responding to the inner call of distress is all that is required of us. Logic and linear reasoning are no help here. Submitting to the struggle begins our healing.

As others acknowledge our plight, we feel a sense of support that gives the time and momentum necessary to move forward to the next stage. A simple acknowledgment from family and health professionals is often the energy necessary to begin to move on.

As we acknowledge the experience, we empower ourselves to merge with it, resonating with the rhythm of the suffering that lies under the physical or emotional pain. After a while we become one with it and recognize its theme.

Here an important shift occurs in our consciousness. Suddenly, as if by magic, we sense a subtle change in perception, sensing a doorway to a new stage of healing. Our total entrapment in consensual reality (a world determined by mass consciousness) is opened as we catch a glimpse into our own subjective intuitive world and the power and wisdom it holds. Feeling raw, disheveled, and very vulnerable, we sense that a barrier has been broken that kept us confined. This moves us to the second stage.

Stage II: Transcending Our Polarities

As we enter this stage, the tendency to judge ourselves and events in our lives intensifies because we now have a "greater I" about ourselves and life around us. Phrases such as "a bad back," or "a lousy situation" abound. We also give ourselves over entirely with blind commitment to the procedures and treatments prescribed by others. However, we also begin to notice that there is a polarity within ourselves. Some parts of our body have a life of their own while others are passive and dependent. Our personality's engagement in judging and evaluating demonstrate that a sense of "me" is developing.

Projection often places the blame outside of ourselves, fostering a danger that may minimize the power of healing insight. Physiologically, we do not have the strength for self-empowerment and so we defer to outside agents easily. Life is experienced as a roller coaster of correcting or being corrected as the polarities create drama in our world and relationships.

Many people get stuck in this stage of healing. Countless self-help courses, books, and diets are consumed by people in this stage. The modern medical establishment and state-of-the-art hospitals are a haven for the cyclical patterns of health-illness in their life. Each encounter, move, or change offers a moment of joy or sense of place, and then, suddenly the pattern repeats. The new job may be worse than the last, the new relationship no more satisfying. The Dalai Lama spoke of this pattern in the dynamic book *Health Through Balance*:

> Basically, every being on this planet—wants happiness and does not want any form of disease or suffering. Yet, we do not know how to achieve the causes of happiness and do not know how to get rid of the causes of suffering.... We make great efforts at techniques for achieving happiness and avoiding pain, but instead, mostly generate just the opposite of what we seek—bringing on ourselves more pain and suffering and diminishing whatever happiness we have. (Dalai Lama, 1986, p. 37)

We discover that what we considered hard and fast rules for good and bad, or right and wrong, become muddled as we begin to realize that what we thought were the roots of our problems were not accurate. We slowly begin to perceive a cyclical pattern in our problems and in our lives. We can begin to recognize a certain pattern in our intimate relationships, as well as those at work and in the larger world.

While the cycle of each being is unique, all cycles fit into an underlying form of the natural rhythm of the universe. From the rise and fall of civilizations to the division of a cell, each cycle fits into the encompassing cadence of earth and cosmos. The Spirit of Universal Consciousness is the timeless wisdom that organizes the universe and also governs the rhythm of our self. Its wisdom is found in our body-mind, guiding us through our own evolution. Disease occurs when we are out of step with our own natural rhythms. Suffering amplifies our natural tendencies, as well as highlighting where the authentic rhythm has been isolated, repressed, or denied. As our strict adherence to rigid rules falls away, we begin to connect more deeply with our own rhythms, and insight grows.

As our insight becomes stronger we quit projecting our problems and ideas onto others, and take them back into ourselves. In this sphere lies the hope for reconciliation of the polarities. We begin to see that instead of life being an endless stream of suffering and drama, it also holds intervals free and open. Our demands, like those of an angry child coming from an unresolved consciousness, give way to requests coming from a more healed and integrated awareness. Occasionally we have a sense of déjà vu, recognizing a repeat of something from the past. We start to notice how our judgments manifest in our life, and we begin to perceive which of our actions trigger specific responses in others. Victim-minded cause and effect gives way to the recognition that we have a role in the process.

As we develop a stronger sense of self, we acquire the strength to assume greater responsibility for our situation. We come to realize that we have been stuck in a perspective while also recognizing that we are responsible for the result. And we become aware of our body holding the imprint of that world-view as blocked energy manifests as an acute or chronic condition. However, while we continually develop a new body-mind, we still persist in manifesting old patterns. Deepak Chopra observed:

> Ninety eight percent of the atoms in our body were not there a year ago. The skeleton that seems so solid was not there a year ago.... The skin is new every month. You have a new stomach lining every four days, with the actual surface cells that contact food being renewed every five minutes. The cells in the liver turn over very slowly, but new atoms still flow through them, like water in a river course, making a new liver every six weeks. (Chopra, 1993, p. 79)

As opposed to organs and soft tissue, nerve cells do not regenerate. It is the nervous system that coordinates consciousness of all body parts, systems, and patterns. This powerful system maintains our body's inner environment, acting as a conduit for the expression of universal consciousness (our inner wisdom). The nervous system establishes who we are and how we interact with the world. When it has not been healed from the trauma of past events, our emotional reality is also stuck. Health, well-being, vitality, and wholeness flow from a nervous system that is free of interference.

Life factors that create interference patterns that are disruptive to the flow of consciousness energy include things such as medications; alcohol; environmental pollutants; chemicals in foods; electromagnetic radiation from computers, cell phones, and appliances; and airplanes. Physical pressure on the nervous system from trauma, tumors, excessive stretching, or twisting and mechanical injury, can also alter the body's ability to heal. Our biography becomes our biology. The combined effects of various stresses and the inability of the nervous system to fully perform its intended functions leads us to being stuck. Pierrakos notes:

> The constrictions of energy ... are not isolated dysfunctions. They are the blocks of stultified energy that trammel the physical body in skeletomuscu-

lar rigidities, and also disrupt the higher planes of energy, thus affecting mental attitudes and expanding consciousness. (Pierrakos, 1987, p. 88)

Epstein (1994, pp. 48–50) observed that with each position of the spine, there is a corresponding predisposition of consciousness, mood, or personality. Being stuck is only partially related to conscious choice, but rather is often a consequence of a fixated nervous system due to a spinal distortion or related problem. Our body movement and tension reveal the history of our physiology, whether we are conscious of it or not.

One of the greatest factors that inhibits healing is the *naming or labeling of a condition*. "You have cancer" gives identification to the issue but immediately prevents us from seeing beyond the assumptions and perceptions about the phenomenon under question. In nursing, the labels affixed to someone or something, whether in charting, giving a shift report, or conversation with patients, families, and coworkers, can be very detrimental to all. Labels give us shortcuts in communication, but often, they also cut short our exchange with the person or phenomena.

Caring for someone at this stage involves offering to assist for a limited period of time until they can figure out how to do things on their own. Such an approach builds a bridge between levels of consciousness that lead to a more expansive perspective. Talking or thinking about a problem does not resolve it, but acknowledging and experiencing it brings it into a personal encounter that can shift perspective. Lowen writes:

> The patient must be brought into touch with reality—the reality of their life situation, the reality of their feelings, and the reality of their body. These three realities cannot be separated from one another. The person who is in touch with their feelings is also in touch with their body situation. By the same logic, the person who is in touch with his body is in touch with all aspects of his life. (Lowen, 1980, pp. 260–261, 267)

Control creates a limited perspective physically, emotionally, mentally, and spiritually, contributing to the perpetuation of the current situation. As the person's sense of self is strengthened, it is time to release efforts to control the chaos, and allow the disruption to more fully impact their life. The more flexible and adaptable the person is, the easier it is to move through this stage. Individuals who are engaged in exercises such as yoga, aerobics, stretching, or athletics move through this stage with a minimum of intervention.

Increasing care options to include holistic practitioners facilitates the healing journey rather than maintaining a continuous focus on controlling symptoms. Flowing through this stage is facilitated by massage therapy, craniosacral and acupuncture therapies, shiatsu and therapeutic touch practitioners, and chiropractors. Healing disciplines such as Jungian therapy, bioenergetics, Healing Touch, Reiki, and Rolfing are other venues that can open the person to new ways of connecting with their body-mind, and moving into the next stage of healing.

Stage III: Moving Towards Authenticity

This stage moves us to reclaiming our personal power while accepting responsibility for our own healing. Key phrases include comments such as, "I'm not going to take this anymore!" or "I must honor who I really am." Here we approach the bifurcation point referred to in quantum physics, where the next path is chosen when we make a choice among the "strange attractors" inviting us forward (Wolf, 1996).

Now we begin to reject our symptoms and separate ourselves from our suffering. Due to our strengthened sense of self, we realize that we have dishonored our inner essence. We decide to step out of suffering, and move in a new direction. This may include leaving a relationship, undergoing surgery, or quitting a job. The other path, chosen less frequently, involves a different state of awareness. Rather than separating from the apparent external cause of our suffering, we assume a greater degree of responsibility for the deeper, less obvious factors that underlie our situation.

Relationships bring about our greatest challenges because we often attract partners who express the alienated aspects of ourselves. Whatever we repress is often expressed by the partner in an intimate relationship, often around issues of work, finances, or relationships. Seeing the patterns of discomfort and struggle as an aspect of life we need to separate from is different than seeing those issues as an expression of interference patterns that are not in sync with the larger rhythms of our life.

This is not a time to decide what to do, but rather a time to work on reclaiming our power. When changes are necessary, our internal wisdom will always guide us. If the path is not clear, it may be that our body-mind has not healed enough to accommodate that change. This juncture is the true beginning of the spiritual journey, as noted by Assagioli:

> Man's spiritual development is a long and arduous journey, an adventure through strange lands full of surprises, difficulties and even dangers. It involves a drastic transformation of the "normal" elements of the personality, an awakening of the potentialities hitherto dormant, a rising of consciousness to new realms, and a functioning alone in a new inner dimension. (Assagioli, 1992, pp. 35–38)

Some will escape the discomfort by producing new patterns in order to control the chaos. Easy ways include finding another partner or avoiding relationships altogether. Changing jobs, seeking therapeutic care from some form of practitioner, psychotherapist, or financial counselor, are all efforts to regain control in their lives. Many people do not complete this stage of the journey.

Quantum physicists have demonstrated that chaos is an essential aspect of life, a necessary ingredient in the evolutionary process. Bohm has observed that

> Chaos science uncovers that the irregularities are not devoid of order; that even seemingly chaotic processes such as weather patterns, and turbulence in fluids is found, on detailed analysis, to exhibit subtle strands of order. (Bohm, 1980, p. 39)

Rather than repressing chaos in our lives, when we have the strength to engage, inviting chaos into our lives gives us the experience and wisdom of its energy. We then discover the lessons nested in the disruptive event as we uncover the underlying order behind its appearance. As disorder strongly impacts our nervous system, our ability to create order out of chaos is a sign of our growing consciousness.

This stage removes all forms of judgment from our lives. Simultaneously, we make a deeper commitment to wholeness in every aspect of our relationship to our reality. Now we gently take our power with no anger or emotional attachment to previous events. We can gaze into a photo album, revisiting the place where our suffering began, and gain insight without emotional storms. We have begun the process of merging with our shadow side.

Here we can observe the process behind our suffering without taking it personally. We look behind the struggle of that event and discover what it has to teach us. We let this process unfold, guided by our inner wisdom rather than our educated minds, with profound results. As we release the emotional attachment to the event, it has a significant nonlocal impact on others also involved in the drama.

As we merge with the illusion of past wounds we feel a new sense of empowerment at the intellectual, spiritual and emotional levels. Blocked energy is released, infusing us with a strength that comes from discovering the truth, opening us to higher dimensions of consciousness energy. We suddenly realize that suffering is not to be taken personally; rather it is a wake-up call to investigate ourselves and our situation more deeply. We begin to understand that in therapy we looked for answers and excuses, while in spiritual healing we seek understanding, and, often, forgiveness.

At this stage a health care practitioner moves from authority figure to partner. What evolves is a practice partnership, where each is committed to the growth, healing, and evolution of the other. The key to healing at this stage is engaging and merging with the issue that fostered the suffering. Resistance to this process occurs as fear of what we imagine may happen overtakes us. As our trusted healing partner asks, "What is the worst that can happen?" we can take the next step. Finding out what lay behind the pattern, knowing what we can do differently and how our lives are to change, can only be understood when we see clearly without illusion. A trusted associate is invaluable to help guide us to the new perspectives on the other side. Completion of this step takes us to the next stage of healing.

Stage IV: Enhancing Capacity

At this stage we are ready to release aspects of ourselves that cannot adapt to our new and stronger sense of self. Trapped perspectives, memories, and energy patterns will be released at the discretion of our inner wisdom, freeing up our body-mind to accommodate an enlarging consciousness. With increased flexibility and momentum we begin to invite change into our life. Larry Dossey notes:

> Health is harmony, and harmony has no meaning without the fluid movement of interdependent parts. Like a stream that becomes stagnant when it ceases to flow, harmony and health turn into disease and death when stasis occurs. We are called to return to the concept of the biodance, the endless streaming of the body-in-flux. (Dossey, 2001, p. 103)

Centering and grounding are the assignments at this stage of healing. We begin to change lifestyle habits, open to new perspectives on healing, and commit to wellness practices. Diet and exercise patterns are reviewed. Activities such as meditation, biofeedback, and yoga are explored. We naturally gravitate towards activities that increase aptitude for movement and awareness, which enhances our capacity for growth and change. At this stage magical synchronicity begins to occur as our body-mind is open and flexible enough to note and accommodate it. Opportunities that align to better our circumstance appear unexpectedly because we are now receptive to them.

A danger at this stage is getting preoccupied with the unfolding process. If we become overly concerned or confused, or doubt our inner wisdom, we may be thrown back to an earlier stage of healing. As we move closer towards discharge of a long-held pattern, uncomfortable feelings are manifest. At this point we may experience nausea, deep sadness, or emotional anxiety, which may foster thoughts of aborting the process. It is imperative that rather than treating the symptoms, we work with a practitioner who can support our further movement into the chaos that is absolutely essential for meaningful change.

Discharge is the precursor to integration. We must accept that we cannot be healthy unless we go out of control through the process of discharging outmoded ways of knowing and being to accommodate our infinite self. Few people allow their body temperature to rise naturally to 102–103 when they are ill. Whenever we interfere with natural body processes, we create more of what our body is trying to eliminate. The discharge will take place when our nervous system is flexible enough to accommodate it.

Symptoms of the discharge process are not a sign of disease, but rather an indication that a healing crisis is moving the body-mind towards resolution and integration. Lack of needed discharge equals lack of health.

Any aspect of our self that no longer works for our best health will be discharged by our innate intelligence. The body-mind will move to eliminate anything, including lifestyle and habits, that no longer serves its highest good. It also discharges the rhythm that cannot live in harmony with the whole. J. Krishnamurti, an Indian philosopher, often taught that to help someone with a problem, all you had to do was understand it without judgment and see it clearly; in time this understanding will be transmitted to the person with the problem. The same holds true for the body.

What many consider as sickness is often the body attempting to discharge or release something it does not want in order to reach a new level of health. After the discharge there is a resolution, much as the relief after a sneeze that produces feelings of calm. A deep sense of accomplishment, freedom, and peace is a sign that integration of the dissonance has occurred with higher order, another movement closer to wholeness.

The discharge process also includes cleaning out closets and desks, going through wardrobes and relationships. It literally is a process of getting one's house in order. We find that we spontaneously release what no longer serves us, making more room and a more flexible system to store material, information, and fresh life experiences that are not simply extensions of the past. This all leads to creation of a fuller experience in the present.

Facilitating this movement towards integration requires us to avoid traps that may derail the process. Old patterns in life revisit us in an effort to bring us back, including: fear of change; self-resentment, which will sabotage the healing process; a personal sense of frustration or deep loneliness; and guilt associated with self-judgment. These feelings prevent us from remaining in the present, drawing us back to earlier stages of our life. Rather than assuming worn-out responses, we simply must be consciously aware of the process that is moving us to the next stage of healing.

Stage V: Emptiness Moving Towards Integration

After discharge is complete, we move towards the moment of emptiness and vulnerability. Much as the crab that has outgrown its shell searches for a new home, we move towards a world of new possibilities with a sense of calm, as well as a knowing that in some ways we are alone. This dynamic sets the stage for deeper exploration and movement forward. We feel raw while we also realize that in a silent space we can tune into the sacred within. We are now without our common reference points that have guided us for years. While it opens new room for possibilities, it is also unsettling. Poet Zambucka wrote:

> And as you reach new plateaus of thought....
> And old friends drop away,
> Fear not loneliness,
> For there is a silent communication between those at the same
> level of awareness.
> And for the first time you will not be lonely....
> (Zambucka, 1984, p. 58)

Emptiness is often confused with nothingness; however, it is so much more than that. It offers a space for transition from one level of consciousness to another, a place to shift the focal point from the lower mind ego of our personality to our higher spiritual ego (Fisher, 1996, pp. 75–78, 95–99). We experience a sense of freedom as our consciousness is not attached to one particular perspective. In the space of emptiness the resonance of our newfound awareness will begin to attract objects, people, and experiences into our world. This empty dynamic state of readiness touches the universal field. Physicist Talbot notes:

> Many physicists believe that at its ultramicroscopic level, empty space is really a turbulent and frothy storm of activity. Moreover ... within these violent upheavals in the nothingness, new particles are constantly being created and destroyed ... ultimately everything we know as real in the entire universe may originally have sprung out of this empty but seething vacuum. (1986, p. 156)

Thus, all potential realities exist in the field of emptiness, which is a state of "everything-ness." Our newfound sense of wholeness and emptiness is a powerful perspective for stepping into the stillness, the place where our own voice can best be heard. We begin to have differing forms of internal dialogue, sensing connections within our self that were not present before. There is a danger at this point to move into ascetic practices that deprive ourselves of various things. However, the stronger response is to honor our inner essence and outer experience through aligning with its natural rhythms.

Practices at this stage involve spontaneous expressions of gratitude. Cultivating a deep sense of appreciation for All-That-Is deepens our connection to the Source. Prayer is another powerful vehicle to express our yearning for relationship and union with the One. Whatever form of religion or spiritual practice one has chosen, prayer waves resonate on the subtle realms of existence, building bridges for healing and grace (Dossey, 1993).

The tone of musical instruments and our own voice facilitate deepening the resonance of our body-mind with the universal rhythms and wholeness of spirit. Yogic practices of rhythmic breath and devotion, chanting and singing, or other forms of gentle movement such as T'ai chi, promote integration. Self-nurturing practices such as massage, a relaxing hot bath, being held by someone else, are all enjoyable and integrating experiences. As we align more closely with our own rhythm, serendipity is a frequent visitor as we resonate more closely with the rhythms of the universe. New and exciting people come into our lives, people who will uplift us, changing our life in positive ways. As we learn to trust the process, and trust ourselves, a deep sense of peace prevails. Derek Walcott invites us:

> The time will come when with elation you will greet yourself,
> Arriving at your own door, in your own mirror,
> And each will smile at the other's welcome;
> Saying, sit here. Eat.
> You will love again the stranger who was yourself.
> Give wine, give bread, give back your heart
> To the stranger who was loved all your life,
> Whom you abandoned for another, who knows you by heart.
> Take down the love letters from the bookshelf, the photographs,
> the desperate notes.
> Sit. Feast on your life.
>
> (Walcott, 2001, p. 5)

The mantra of the day becomes simply, thank you, as you move into the next stage of healing.

Stage VI: Shifting the Focal Point

As we begin to move within this higher state of conscious awareness, we begin to perceive that life is more than an outward physical manifestation. We can literally see and feel the true essence of existence; energy, form, and the light behind form. We begin to perceive the life force of energy as an intelligence flowing through us. It appears as warmth, vitality, light, color and sound, or a tingling sensation.

For the first time we experience ourselves as part of a larger reality, one comprised of energy rather than physical things. We begin to relate to life beyond physical form, experiencing the beauty, excitement, and joyful vitality found in the natural world, and in all things. Redfield provides insight to this phenomenon:

> We humans will learn to perceive what was formerly invisible types of energy.... Human perception of this energy first begins with a heightened sensitivity to beauty ... the perception of beauty is a kind of barometer telling each of us how close we are to actually perceiving this energy. (Redfield, 1993, p. 17)

Gratitude and acknowledgement of the flow of life, as opposed to manipulation and control, are signs that ego investment has been transcended. We do not need to change anything, but rather, be in harmony with the stage we are in, whether for ourselves or others. Epstein has observed that "expecting and honoring what is observed is enough for it to be transformed on its own accord" (1994, pp. 183–186).

At this stage, thoughts begin to break up from patterned thinking to energy packets of attention. Fresh awareness and understanding emerge as we work through the higher intelligence of spiritual ego, accompanied with feelings of joy, gratitude, and love that allow for accommodation of our spirituality and wholeness. Suddenly we are "no one" as our old forms begin to dissolve. We begin to separate from the rest of the world, merging increasingly with the unrecognized wholeness of our being. Here we feel safe, connected, embraced, and embracing. We are both observing ourselves and experiencing ourselves beyond all boundaries as polarity has been transcended. Parmahansa Yogananda, the beloved teacher of Kriya Yoga, taught that divine energy flow and connection with the Ultimate One is experienced in eight ways: light, sound, peace, calmness, love, joy, wisdom, and power (Yogananda, 1959). Here there is no sense of separation and everything we touch enriches us. As with every other stage, surrendering fully to the moment empowers us to move to the next stage.

Stage VII: Returning to Community

We move back into connection with ordinary reality knowing that the source of love and power is enfolded in universal consciousness. It does not come from, nor does it depend upon us. This gift from the One is available to all. That knowing transforms the life we continue to live going forward in a more loving and compassionate way. Meditation teacher Jack Kornfield observed:

> You have to live your spirituality day to day, at home, at work, in your car. Otherwise, it won't transform you, and in the end you won't benefit and transform the world around you. (Kornfield, 1993, p. 116)

Our expanded world is filled with more energy, a broader perspective, and greater understanding. We naturally align with life's natural rhythms, serving as conduits for the universal rhythms, uplifting situations around us as we no longer engage in the drama. Our daily practice includes remaining mindful of the miracle of life, and expressing gratitude for its generous gifts. We make a deeper commitment to being a healing presence in the world. Trungpa observed:

> You can invoke and provoke the uplifted energy of basic goodness in your life. You begin to see how you can create basic goodness for yourself and others on the spot, fully and ideally, not only on a philosophical level, but on a concrete physical level. (Trungpa, 1984, p. 85)

People and experiences continue to emerge that invite us to liberate ourselves from old perspectives, furthering our growth. We begin to recognize that our thoughts are distractions—concepts, comparisons, and analysis are habits that prevent focus on the moment and what is trying to occur. We have come to understand that healing occurs in the moment, which is also the eternal. Chopra addresses timeless awareness:

> Healing comes about through transcendence. There is no other way out. To see things with the crystal clarity of pure awareness not through the old memories, not remaining a victim of the stale repetition of old memories. So we reexperience pain, sorrow, anger, guilt, physical conditions with this new awareness, no longer being attached to them, observing them, observing ourselves, observing the action. (Chopra, 1993, p. 43)

As things are viewed from a larger vantage, we experience love with no conditions. We no longer care if our ideas or offerings are well received; we simply submit them as an authentic gift from the heart. As we become more open and available to others, our sense of community increases.

We begin to see community in everything from the cells that support our body to the cosmic sky. In community, we find places within ourselves where we had lost our participation. We now have healed sufficiently to share our gifts of wisdom, understanding, and compassion, which were acquired on our healing journey. Sharing our wounds is a sacred act, for they contain the seeds of healing for both ourselves and the universe.

Healing is a lifelong process, one that is part of our task while living on Earth, our home for evolution, learning, and service. Bailey described this healing presence:

> When man functions as a soul, he heals; he stimulates and vitalizes; he transmits the spiritual forces of the universe.... Humanity's function is to transmit and handle force. This is done in the early and ignorant stages destructively and with harmful results. Later, when acting under the influence of the soul, force is rightly and wisely handled ... more mercifully. Wholeness is its outcome. (Bailey, 1970, p. 99)

As we support others with a spirit of compassion, the hallmark of nursing, we connect through our shared quality of love. Love is movement out of stillness, the movement of evolution. In this space we foster sharing, unfolding, flowering, and becoming whole. Nursing gives us a vehicle to express these qualities, a way to share the energy of unconditional regard. Sharing is the ultimate movement of community, and only a world of sharing can be a peaceful and healthy world.

> *Patience is not waiting passively for something to happen, but is a kind of participation with the other in which we give fully of ourselves. It is misleading to understand patience simply in terms of time, for we give the other space as well. By patiently listening to the distraught person, by being present for them, we give them space to think and feel. Perhaps, instead of speaking of space and time, it would be truer to say that the patient person gives the other room to live; they enlarge the other's living room, whereas the impatient person narrows it.*
>
> Milton Mayeroff

BIBLIOGRAPHY

Assagioli, R. (1992). *Psychosynthesis.* New York: Anchor.

Bailey, A. A. (1970). *A treatise on white magic.* New York: Lucis.

Bendit, L. J. (1973). *The mysteries today.* London: The Theosophical Publishing House.

Bohm, D. (1980). *Wholeness and the implicate order.* London: Routledge and Kegan Paul.

Chopra, D. (1989). *Quantum healing.* New York: Bantam.

Chopra, D. (1993). *Ageless mind, timeless body.* New York: Harmony.

Dalai Lama. (1986). *Health through balance.* Ithaca, NY: Snow Lion.

Dossey, L. (1993). *Healing words: The power of prayer and the practice of medicine.* New York: HarperCollins.

Dossey, L. (2001). *Healing beyond the body.* Boston: Shambhala.

Epstein, D. M. (1994). *The 12 stages of healing: A network approach to wholeness.* San Rafael, CA: Amber-Allen.

Fisher, B. S. (1996). *Man, grand reflection of the greater cosmos: Studies in occult anatomy.* (Vol. 3). Prescott, AZ: Subru.

Goswami, A. (2004). *The quantum doctor: A physicist's guide to health and healing.* Charlottesville, VA: Hampton Roads.

Kornfield, J. (1993). *A path with heart: A guide through the perils and promises of spiritual life.* New York: Bantam.

Lowen, A. (1980). *Depression and the body.* New York: Pelican.

Osho. (2003). *Mind-body balancing: Using your mind to heal your body.* New York: St. Martin's Griffin.

Pierrakos, J. (1987). *Core energetics.* Mendocino, CA: LifeRhythm.

Prigogine, I. (1976). Order through fluctuation: Self-organization and social system. In E. J. Jantsch & C. H. Waddington (Eds.), *Evolution and consciousness* (pp. 93–133). Reading, MA: Addison-Wesley.

Redfield, J. (1993). *The celestine prophecy.* Hoover, AL: Satori.

Roberts, B. (1985). *The path to no-self.* Boston: Shambhala.

Schoch, M. (2005). *Healing with qualities.* Boulder, CO: Sentient.

Talbot, M. (1986). *Beyond the quantum.* New York: Macmillian.

Trungpa, C. (1984). *The sacred path of the warrior.* Boston: Shambhala.

Walcott, D. (2001). *Uses of enchantment.* New York: Vintage.

Wolf, F. A. (1996). *The spiritual universe.* New York: Simon and Schuster.

Yogananda, P. (1959). *Whispers for eternity.* Los Angles: Self-Realization Fellowship.

Zambucka, K. (1984). *The keepers of the Earth.* Honolulu, HI: Harrame.

CHAPTER 7

Healing Presence

The Path of Engagement

Do not think that love, in order to be genuine, has to be extraordinary.
What we need is to love without getting tired.
How does a lamp burn? Through the continuous input of small drops of oil.
If the drops of oil run out, the light of the lamp will cease....
My daughters, what are these drops of oil in our lamps?
They are the small things of daily life;
faithfulness, punctuality, small words of kindness, a thought for others,
our way of being silent, of looking, of speaking, and of acting.
These are the true drops of love....
Be faithful in small things because it is in them that your strength lies.

Mother Teresa

Many things in life matter, but only one thing really matters absolutely. It matters whether we succeed or fail in the eyes of the world. It matters whether we are healthy or not, whether we are educated or not, it matters if we are rich or poor—that certainly makes a difference in how our lives unfold. While all of these things matter, relatively speaking, they do not matter absolutely.

There is one thing that matters more than any of those things; it is finding the essence of who we are beyond the short-lived personalized sense of self. For when we are aligned with the innate rhythms and patterns of our life we are in harmony with All-That-Is. Peace is not found in rearranging the circumstances of our life, but, rather, by realizing who we are at the deepest level of our soul (Tolle, 2003).

We are born with an insatiable curiosity and desire to learn; an instinctive search for our soul. Unfortunately, learning is often seen as a process of analyzing mistakes and modifying behavior based on those experiences. Real learning, however, involves an experiment, experiencing the outcome

115

and leaving it at that; simply forgetting it and moving forward. When a baby tries to stand but keeps falling over, it does not sit down and analyze what occurred, judging if it tried hard enough. It just keeps trying over and over again, making minor adjustments in balance until, at last, the desired outcome appears.

Subtle energy follows thought. The moment we start judging our learning, our energy gets diverted into questioning our progress. Learning involves cycles of experimentation and forgetting. Forgetting means to learn without judging or focusing on our perceived weaknesses and mistakes. In true learning there are no mistakes, only steps in an unfolding journey of discovery. Fixating on our weaknesses diverts energy and focus, creating unnecessary problems and lack of freedom.

Where there is no freedom there is security; the opposite of security is not insecurity, but freedom. Learning is the movement of stepping into a new space where we are totally insecure about what will happen next. Studies have shown that when children are faced with a choice between an intriguing learning situation and restraint from a parent, they will choose the learning experience. Not because they don't love their parents, but because biological consciousness, curiosity, is stronger than love. It involves being totally ready to move outward, away from safety, even if it jeopardizes one's own life. Such is the intelligence of evolution: consciousness is not possible without curiosity and learning (Schoch, 2005, p. 18). It is this kind of evolutionary learning that is facing nursing in the postmodern world.

Health care in the twenty-first century will require a radically different practitioner, a nurse who must transcend the caring model that has been practiced since the discipline's inception. In her pathbreaking work, *Postmodern Nursing and Beyond,* nurse theorist Jean Watson (1999) addresses the changing landscape of health care in general, and nursing specifically. She identifies the need for nursing not only to embrace a new health care paradigm that honors the feminine, but also to adopt an ontological shift of a deeper nature.

This evolutionary shift in perspective acknowledges the emerging symbiotic relationship between humankind-technology-nature and the larger, expanding universe. Declaring that a sea-change of such magnitude is evoking a return to the sacred core of humanity, she invites nurses to develop a transpersonal caring focus in their practice.

> Transpersonal conveys a human connection, beyond personal body-physical ego, and has a spiritual dimension; it implies a focus on the uniqueness of self and other coming together, moving from the fully embodied physical ego-self to deeper, more spiritual, transcendent even cosmic connections that tap into healing; transpersonal includes the unique individuality of each human, while extending beyond the ego-self, radiating and transcending to

deeper connections all humans share with their deeper selves, the other, environment, nature and the universe. (Watson, 1999, pp. 290–291)

Transpersonal caring is a founding construct for the essence of a healing presence. This stance will bring nursing from the modern into the postmodern era, giving us the opportunity to reinstate the sacred feminine into the healing arts. Restoring the masculine-feminine balance will return the possibility for wholeness into the healing experience. As all health care workers incorporate methods that work directly with cycle, rhythm, resonance, reciprocity, and right relationship—the patterns of the feminine—the power of the self to heal will be potentiated. Respect, integrity, and compassion will be restored into the healing relationship. This will give the diverse assemblage of healing practitioners an equal place in cooperative and collaborative practice models. However, it will require the development of new ways of seeing, knowing, and being.

SPIRITUAL DIMENSIONS OF NURSING: PRESENCE AND WISDOM

From a stance of reverence and openness towards the limitless possibilities in both inner and outer space, we may bring the spiritual aspects of our being into our nursing practice, and our relationships with all. Before we can offer such a perspective to others, we must first cultivate this consciousness within ourselves.

In their compelling book *The Spirituality of Imperfection,* Kurtz and Ketcham compare the discovery of spirituality to playing baseball, the only sport that considers errors to be an integral part of the game:

> Spirituality teaches us, or has taught most of us, how to deal with failure. We learn at a very young age that failure is the norm in life...errors are part of the game, part of its rigorous truth. (Kurtz & Ketcham, 1992, p. 1)

For thousands of years, everyday saints and mystics have explored the ordinary and common in an attempt to understand the extraordinary and divine. Their various attempts call forth the spiritual realities of humility, gratitude, tolerance, and forgiveness. The spirituality of imperfection begins with the recognition that trying to be perfect is the most tragic human mistake. When we cease trying to be perfect, by embracing our errors and shortcomings and accepting that we cannot control every aspect of our lives, we begin to find peace and serenity, and the joy of our authentic selves.

The call for a transpersonal awareness is not a call to sainthood; it is a call to authenticity. For us individually, and nursing as a collective, to move deeper into our own being and then extending it as an offering to others requires the courage to see the truth of what is, to be totally present, to simply observe what is there and establish a relationship with it. We will discover that within ourselves, and in each human being, there is a dimension of consciousness far deeper than thought; it is the *essence of who we are*. It has been referred to as many things, including presence, awareness, unconditional consciousness, the Christ within, or your Buddha nature.

Finding that dimension frees us, and the world, from the suffering that we inflict upon ourselves through the countless little judgments made by the mind's ego that runs our lives. Love, peace, and creativity cannot come into our lives while that unconditioned dimension of consciousness dominates. When we step out of the content of our lower mind, the incessant stream of thinking slows down. Thoughts do not absorb all of our attention anymore. Gaps arise in between thoughts—spaciousness—stillness. In the silence we begin to realize how much vaster and deeper we are than our thoughts.

As our self-awareness grows, we can recognize, even for a second, that the thoughts running through our mind are simply thoughts, habits, and patterns that do nothing except divert our attention and energy towards maintaining the status quo. The human mind, with its curious drive to know, understand, and control, mistakes its own opinions and viewpoints as the truth. It continually tells us "this is how it is," and we believe it.

Expanded consciousness, our spiritual ego, which is larger than thought, helps us to realize that no matter how we interpret our life or the life or behavior of another, it's no more than a point of view, one of many possible perspectives. Thinking fragments reality into conceptual bits and pieces. But the perspective of soul sees the truth that reality is one beautiful and unified whole, in which all things are interwoven, and nothing exists alone. From a stance of unconditional regard, we sense the union and security of being part of All-That-Is, fostering a sense of safety and peace beyond understanding. Only when we are in this loving space of oneness with all will true wisdom emerge as we see and understand holistically.

As professionals we have been socialized to utilize a highly sophisticated conceptually oriented and analytical mind. While this is a very useful and powerful tool, it also is very limiting when it overtakes our larger perspective, when we quit realizing that it is only one small aspect of the wisdom in higher consciousness that we are.

Awareness creates the context of active receptivity, an essential aspect of a healing presence. A nurse who is authentically present moves between the world of clinical practice (figure) and the context of the person's life (ground), weaving an invisible web of interconnection between the immediate and the important, between the visible and the invisible, between endings and beginnings, between despair and renewal. It is this vibrant space of all possibility that gives the person perspective, hope, and direction for the life that is emerging out of the chaos of the moment.

To see and respond to the invisible half of wholeness, nursing must expand its capacity in all three domains: the science, the art, and the essence of their practice. The evaluator aspect of the nurse as scientist must develop the mechanisms of active observation. The interpreter aspect of the nurse as artist must increase skills in active intelligence. And, the witness aspect of the essence of the nurse must increase the capacity to create and maintain a context of active receptivity, the space that integrates all with spiritual ego. Building on the strong framework for practice, which is our heritage, we must now make the quantum leap into a new dimension if we are to honor our social commitment to the public we are privileged to serve.

The notion of being active implies an awareness coming from a place beyond the thinking mind. Judgment and labels, prejudice of any kind, implies that we are identified with the thinking mind. It means that we do not see the other human being any longer, only our predetermined concept of that person. To reduce the aliveness of another to a concept is a form of violence.

Thinking that is not rooted in awareness becomes self-serving and dysfunctional. Intelligence devoid of wisdom is extremely dangerous and destructive (as seen in the prevalence of war in today's society). Focus coming from the thinking mind is the current state of mass consciousness in humanity. The amplification of thought as science and technology, though not intrinsically good or bad, has become destructive because so often the thinking out of which it arises has no roots in awareness.

Nursing in the postmodern world must move from thinking to the stance of wisdom. Wisdom is not a product of thought. The deep *knowing* that is wisdom arises through the simple act of giving someone or something your full attention. Attention is primordial intelligence; consciousness itself. This powerful awareness dissolves the barriers created by conceptual thought, and with this comes the recognition that nothing exists by itself. It joins the perceiver and that which is perceived into a unified field of awareness (Tolle, 2003, p. 16). *It is the energy of conscious awareness that is invited and honored through a healing presence.*

ACTIVE OBSERVATION: SEEING BEYOND THE OBVIOUS

Physical assessment is the starting point for nursing practice. Once the therapeutic relationship is established, the task set before the nurse is to evaluate the phenomenon at hand from an objective stance and then create a plan of care. The patient experience is dictated by the depth and breadth of the assumptions, observations, and conclusions drawn about their situation. Addressing patient care needs will include only the things that our awareness and understanding can recognize. The patient is at the mercy of the nurse.

Our current professional education curriculum focus has been on physical assessment, evaluating the status of the body and the emotional/spiritual well-being of the person entrusted to our care. In the postmodern world an expanded approach is required of the nurse-healer. We must move from physical assessment (object assessment) to undivided assessment (object and field assessment). Simultaneously, we are asked to move from focused intervention to a nonintervention focus that facilitates cocreation of a healing strategy with the person.

- *Active Observation:* Moving from concrete thought to the active stance of observation requires the development of capacity to assess both the tangible and the subtle. It also requires us to enter the experience from a perspective of relationship rather than an interventional viewpoint.
- *Undivided Assessment:* In undivided assessment we evaluate and sense the energetic field just as we evaluate physical/concrete reality. This requires us to expand our sense capacity for hearing and looking with a new sense ability of listening and seeing in our evaluative role.

In the quantum world we utilize both a passive mechanism of looking and an active mechanism of seeing to comprehend the whole of the situation under review. The nurse evaluator will utilize five instruments of sight:

- the eye—the organ of sight
- the brain—the organ of transfer
- the concrete lower mind—which discriminates and sorts out the signals from the first two
- the abstract upper mind—which evaluates the information transmitted by the lower mind, translating it into pattern recognition
- the intuition—the sense of "I" or inner wisdom that holds the collective wisdom of all of our lives' experiences

Together these five components constitute the "Internal Instrument," which serves as a link between the body-mind-ego embedded in our personality and the spiritual ego that resides in our soul. There are two mechanisms used to create integrated vision (Fisher, 1996, pp. 49–53):

- *A Passive Mechanism:* energy patterns in the form of light and etheric atoms emanate from the object to be perceived. Light carries information about its form, focused by refracting media onto the retina of the physical eye. This pattern is transmitted by light-sensitive cells (rods and cones) via the optic nerve onto the physical brain.

Ordinary sight (physical vision) is based upon highly organized and localized organs of perception, specialized from chemical and etheric physical matter. This organic process helps us to see in the traditional sense of sight.

- *An Active Mechanism:* likened to a radar system. An energy beam emitted by the optic nerve illuminates and penetrates the object to be perceived, mingles with the energy patterns emitted by the object as interference patterns meet, and is reflected back and focused on the etheric lens of the third eye. The energy pattern carried is impressed directly upon the optic disc and transmitted via the optic nerve onto the physical brain.

Perception (mental vision) is less localized and more symmetrically distributed over the ovoid surface of the emotional body and mental body auras. They each contain force-centers or vortices that function as receptors for perception of energy patterns. However, the circulation is so rapid, as is the interchange between the substances of the emotional and mental worlds that perception is virtually with these bodies-as-a-whole, in holographic fashion. This gives us a sense-perception of an invisible whole behind the specific object viewed by the third eye.

Along with visual assessment, we utilize auditory sound to deepen our understanding; we tune in to the stereo sound that informs a deeper knowing. When we casually focus our attention on what is being said we hear the message of the words. However, when we listen with full attention, our thought body senses the energetic tone, holographically perceiving the message behind the words. Giving ourselves completely to the act of listening beyond the sounds uncovers something greater, a sacredness that cannot be understood through thought (Tolle, 1999, p. 77).

Full understanding occurs in the silence. We become aware of awareness as the background to all of our thoughts and perceptions. The formless dimension of pure consciousness arises from within us and replaces identification with concepts and preformed ideas. True intelligence operates silently. Stillness is where insight, creativity, and solutions to problems are found.

A healing presence is truly open to a situation with nonjudgment and nonexpectancy. In actively seeing and hearing a picture of the whole, the seen and the unseen, the object and the ground will emerge. If we come with a preconceived idea of what should be present, we will find only what we are looking for, or its absence. Developing the capacity for object and ground perception with an open mind occurs as we move beyond labels and judgment.

- *Nonintervention:* We are called to move from beginning the nurse-patient connection with a diagnosis and intervention focus, to coming into the relationship with no-mind. When we place a label on a person or situation we confuse the conditioned mind maps and plans with the truth of what is before us. To function in this way is an unconscious pattern, deeply conditioned through childhood, and cultural and professional socialization. Once we place a conceptual identity on something it becomes a prison for both the other and for ourselves.

The curing paradigm is prescriptive, requiring the practitioner to identify what is wrong and take steps to fix it. When health is viewed as a disruption in multiple levels of energy/consciousness, the approach of treating a person with a specific intervention becomes a problem. Physician Rachel Naomi Remen observed:

> The curing relationship is not always healthy for the client. While benefiting in some ways by the relationship, the client may also be diminished because it is a dependent relationship. There is not much room for strength or growth in the kind of curing relationship that we're taught in professional schools. We can fix the fixable, direct and control specific outcomes, but we don't evoke healing, and we don't participate in the healing that may arise naturally. The fixing relation assumes that healing occurs naturally, following its own natural course. This is wrong and the outcome is often incomplete. (Quoted in Kuthumi, 1996, p. 158)

We are called to move from an intervention-driven practice into *the realm of nonintervention.* We cannot know what form the multidimensional pattern of a person will take as their awareness expands. The new paradigm that focuses on healing is relational. The nurse and patient enter into a partnership, an authentic relationship where both persons trust the process that evolves. This requires nurses to bring their awareness and presence, rather than their doing, as the *primary* mechanism for helping. Of course, the science and interventions of professional practice are always there, but they reside in the background, waiting to be called upon, rather than in the foreground controlling what is trying to emerge.

> Placing nursing/caring into a spiritual perspective in no way diminishes what we have to offer others through training, experience, individuality, special skills, or sense of human. Quite the reverse. Our particular talents and unique qualities are likely to come forth more reliably when we do have a richer and more spacious sense of who we are—the very promise of all spiritual practice. (Ram Dass)

Non-intervention is based on a holographic model of wave interference. Concentric rings of light-energy are consistently emanating from every living thing. In the human they originate in the heart chakra, primarily, and other chakras secondarily (Djwal Kul, 1996). See Figure 7.1.

Each person has a specific wave pattern, the reflection of their personality and four lower bodies in the concrete world. Energy waves are holographic in nature, with the image of the whole written on each part.

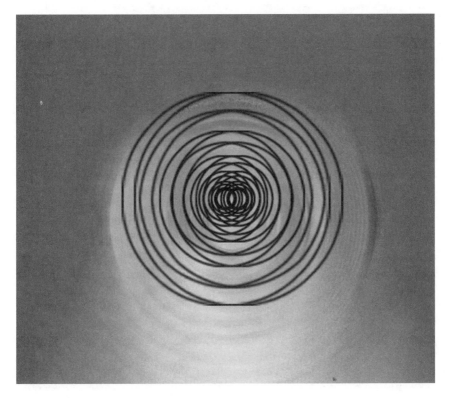

FIGURE 7.1   Concentric rings emanating from chakras.

Just as waves emerge from two pebbles tossed into water, energy waves are emitted from two people in close proximity. As the waves radiate toward each other, they meet and interact and an interference pattern evolves. The pattern spreads and is part of the whole of the previous patterns. To be in touch with the other person and the environment, one must be in touch with their own pattern. Research shows that when two people were focusing on each other in a meaningful way, their EEG patterns merged as one. Our ability to pick up signals increases during a deep interpersonal connection. Braud's research further demonstrated that the most ordered brain pattern always prevailed. Mental and physical structures of a highly organized person exerted an ordering influence on the less-organized recipient (Braud, 2000). See Figure 7.2.

The patient and nurse are interpenetrating aspects of a shared whole. The unbroken wholeness of the partnership is also part of the universal energy field, as the holographic view of the world is enfolded in each region of space-time. In nested hierarchy, individual pattern is contained within our own orb, while in a shared space we become part of another. On the universal level, we are part of All-That-Is. The order recorded in the complex movement of these

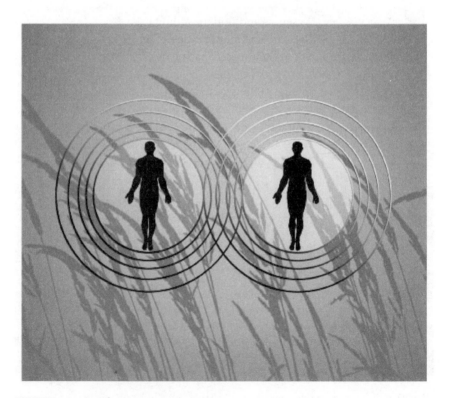

FIGURE 7.2   Interference patterns between two persons.

electromagnetic fields enfolds the entire information of the universe in each region of space and time (Bohm, 1981). The clearer we know ourselves, the more clear we are in knowing other persons, and the more meaningful will be our relationships. The highest form of knowing is love, the essence of the Spirit of Universal Consciousness.

Traditional nursing practice utilized the scientific process of assessment, diagnosis, intervention, and evaluation. The relational paradigm utilizes the process of pattern recognition; exchanging, communicating, relating, valuing, choosing, moving, perceiving, feeling, and knowing (Madrid & Barrett, 1994; Newman, 1986; Parse, 1995; Watson, 1999). Inductive clustering of information coupled with deductive selection of crucial concepts guides the nurse's clinical reasoning process (Pesut & Hermann, 1999).

When we give our full attention to the present moment and what we are interacting with, we take past and future out of the relationship, except for practical matters. Immediate and emergent conditions always demand a swift response. However, as we relinquish conditioned expectations and reactions, attention steps in and shows us a deeper truth, making the resulting intervention more profound and therapeutic. In the process both the nurse and the person increase their awareness and understanding from the unique perspective that is their own. Both become more in the exchange but in different and unique ways appropriate for their own capacity, rather than in a scripted and predetermined fashion.

There is a clear distinction between motivative thinking (descriptive, analytic, and intelligent thought, which is the first part of the thought process), and associative thinking (secondary thought creating a mental picture of the future and anything negative that might happen). Active awareness requires us to be constantly attentive to our thoughts and our relationship to them. The following principles assist us in shifting to a new way of observing and thinking with awareness (Schoch, 2005, p. 67):

- Know that you can understand and at the same time be aware of how your thought processes work.
- Use your motivative thinking to become aware of the associative thinking process so that you can influence your associative thoughts.
- Always be aware of your inner dialogue, the description that is running constantly in your head.
- Be aware of how you build up description in associative thoughts as you focus on what you desire to be different, better, more loved, more powerful, or perfect.
- Stop analyzing problems. Look at them directly without asking why. Inquire as to how you might solve them and move forward.

- When searching for a solution to a problem choose the most practical one. If you tend to go for the most difficult solution, it shows how your thinking is trapped in the descriptive process of wanting perfection. When you take a simple and practical approach, the associative thought process is not activated.
- Ask yourself if you are ready to examine your belief systems and if necessary let them go. Realize that 80% of the ego is identified with belief systems, theoretical structures, habits, and rituals.

As we develop a connection with our thoughts, we establish a consistent relationship with them. This moves us from thinking as the constant evaluator to a more neutral position of the observer, the function of the higher mind.

ACTIVE INTELLIGENCE: KNOWING BEYOND CONCRETE THOUGHT

In the postmodern world an expanded approach to thought is required of the nurse-healer. We must move from concrete thinking (logic, analysis, and understanding) to a higher perspective of active intelligence that also incorporates abstract thinking (intuition, intent, and wisdom). Simultaneously, we are asked to shift the focal point of thought from the lower dimension of body-mind-ego to the higher dimension of the spiritual ego, which increases vibrational energy and access to our inner wisdom as well as universal intelligence.

Active Intelligence: A nurse-healer in the postmodern world utilizes new models for discernment that transcend understanding, expanding the scholarly practice of their trade. To efficiently do this we are called to shift our focal point, the point of awareness, to the higher realm of abstract thought. Exploring current models of logic and the classical metaphysical archetypes, we come to understand a way of knowing that transcends our current knowledge systems. See Figure 7.3.

Energy follows subtle thought. Our thoughts, which create our world, emerge from the universal energy field existing as the pure energy of universal intelligence. The home of the human mind is our thought world, comprised of seven levels that are divided into two regions and a transitional mid-level (Fisher, 1996, pp. 49–53):

- The region of concrete thought consists of the three lower levels of body-mind whose force-matter is of sufficiently low vibrational rate that it may be molded into thought-forms. Three levels of embodied thought are manifest in the gross physical body as

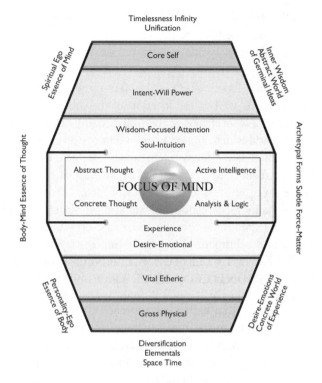

FIGURE 7.3   Body, Mind and Spirit.

- senses (vital etheric)
- feelings (desire emotional)
- analysis and logic (the lower three levels of the mental reflective body)

This is the home of the personality and ego; our common sense. *Experience is the gateway into our body-mind, or concrete self.*

- The region of abstract thought consists of the three upper levels of spiritual consciousness, whose energy is of such high vibrational rate that it cannot be molded into form. Rather, it serves as the medium for germinal ideas. The three levels of higher consciousness include
  - wisdom (focused intuition)
  - intent (will-power)
  - your core *self* (the originating spark of your specific life, which is a direct extension of the Source)

The region of abstract thought is home to the spiritual ego, our higher self, which contains all love-wisdom acquired across all previous life experiences. *Active intelligence is the gateway into our abstract self.*

- The mid-level (fourth level) of the thought world is the *home of the human mind,* as well as the location of the focus of mind, which is the *focal point of awareness* of the individual. Its exact location in the thought world is determined by the vibratory level of the person and can be shifted as we develop our capacity for active intelligence. It is called the region of archetypal forces, because at this level germinal ideas begin to impress as archetypes of form. Universal energy converts to vitality globules for the vital and physical body. Personality's desires and emotional thought forms are crystallized to reflect the cravings and sentiment of the body-mind, triggering receptor proteins in the cells. Simultaneously, pondering abstract ideas or aesthetic thoughts and emotions directs the subtle universal energy upwards towards the region of abstract thought, strengthening inner wisdom and the spiritual ego.
- The mental body-mind is an organized cloud of force-matter specialized from the region of concrete thought. Ovoid in shape, it encircles the physical/vital and emotional bodies, vibrating at two levels, which serve as a bridge between the regions of concrete and abstract thought.
  - Its sector of lower vibration serves as our organ of *concrete thought,* our vehicle for thinking. Because of predominant thinking patterns, the focal point directs most of the mental body's matter to the brain in the physical body, which records the ongoing thoughts and emotions of the personality; the "i". A diffused and less conditioned consciousness, it creates a small "envelope" identified strongly with our emotions and ego. Focusing on this dimension of awareness limits capacity and options, and we easily get entangled in the external world. This aspect of concrete mind predominates in most people today; it is mass consciousness.
  - Its sector of higher vibration serves as a vehicle for *abstract thought,* the seat of the intuitive mind and higher intellect; the "I". It serves as the doorway into the abstract world of the spiritual ego. It is also the portal through which creative, germinal ideas flow from the field of infinite possibility.
  - The *home of the soul,* our individuality, intuition, and conscience is found within the sector of higher vibration located in the sixth dimension directly over the heart chakra. When the focal point

shifts into the domain of active intelligence, the mental body's matter begins to move into the world of abstract thought. The soul increasingly contributes aspects of our unique potential and specific information that guides our life purpose into the reality we are creating. This increased vibrational shift and information from our inner wisdom initiates synchronicity into our life.

The concrete world is still available, but the initiating thoughts begin at a higher, more abstract level of consciousness. From this perspective, an active, versus. prescriptive, intelligence navigates multiple dimensions and opens-limitless possibilities. In this world we cocreate reality rather than conform to it.

Just as water can appear as solid, liquid, or gas, consciousness also changes form. It can be seen as frozen (essence of body) in physical matter, the outcome of concrete thought. Consciousness can also be viewed as liquid (essence of being) when force-matter is forming in the thought world, guided by either the direction of our declared intent (will-power) or the desires of the personality (emotions). Then there is a formless source of consciousness (essence of divine) in the abstract world of the spiritual ego. Pure consciousness emanates from the universal field, the Source as pure energy, pure consciousness, pure love, before it comes into manifestation. The world we create is a reflection of our level of consciousness.

Thought has great creative power; it is the creative force in the universe. Creativity is a specialized way of thinking. Situational creativity, rearrangement of things that exist, is utilized as we work through issues and opportunities on a daily basis. Foundational creativity, however, is more rare and difficult. The domain of artists, adepts, and cultural creatives, it involves the creation of new order, whether in form, the written word, or social order.

The creative act begins with intent. Don Juan instructed Carlos Castaneda with these words:

> In the universe there is an immeasurable, indescribable force which shamans call intent, and absolutely everything that exists in the entire cosmos is attached to intent by a connecting link. When those who live with the source beckon with intent, it comes to them and sets up the path for attainment, which means they always accomplish what they set out to do. (Castaneda, 1972, p. 3)

The field of intent is guided energy from the universe. Nonlocal and ubiquitous, it is everywhere. This invisible and formless field is manifest in every part of our body, our soul, and the reality we create. It is the subtle pull towards the potential for the purpose of our life prompted by our spiritual ego (Woody, 2004, p. 59). When personality ego dominates, however, the power of intent is disconnected, and we become passive, living in reactive fashion in the world of our persona.

Conversely, when intent is resolute, a sincere act of will emanating from the highest aspect of our spiritual ego, it calls forth a concept or germinal idea that moves into the region of our thought world. Here the thought-form attracts force matter to create a "desire element," which will impel action in the physical world.

We may request one thing yet experience something quite different from our expectations because manifestation occurs in relation to our vibrational capacity. Thought forms follow the subtle energy patterns that radiate from our body-mind. A neutral force, they are without judgment. They honor what we are thinking about, not what we are talking about. It is the desire/emotional body patterns that create the form of our reality. Fear and anger are two vibrational energetic patterns that most often sabotage the longings of our heart.

Nurse-healers can expand their mental body-mind and capacity for active intelligence through disciplines of logic such as studying the new physical quantum sciences and mathematics. Focusing on artistic expressions of music and poetry, photography, and stories increases sensitivity to the universal in all things. Aesthetic creative activities and noble ideas and acts of compassion increase the capacity for love-wisdom. Flexibility and adaptability increase through the practice of various forms of body work. And we can become infinitely more responsive to the subtle promptings of our body-mind-spirit by managing emotions or cultivating the art of stillness through meditation and awareness practices.

Shifting the focal point requires raising the vibrations of the mental body, making it more luminous, organizing it into a more definitive structure, and freeing it from the influences of desire and emotions. This will make it invulnerable to the negative and destructive thought-forms and desires created by others. They abound in the environment, and are often assimilated by us, manifesting similar destructive tendencies in ourselves. As we move the focus of our mental body towards our higher intelligence, increasing amounts of force-matter will shift from the brain in the lower body into the abstract realm. Our thought patterns will move to a higher dimension, opening us up to a new knowledge that transcends thought and understanding.

Our personality traits and patterns are the external manifestation of our inner world; consciousness is who we are (Tolle, 2005). As our understanding of that grows, we begin to see ourselves in everything. The heavy screen of past, concepts, and attitudes through which all things are filtered drops away. We begin to perceive without interpreting. From the realm of higher consciousness we can perceive the essence of what we observe. Michelangelo remarked that "every beauty which is seen here below by persons of perception resembles more than anything else that celestial source from which we all came" (quoted in Dwyer, 2004, p. 1). Increasingly we become that which we appreciate, and our healing presence unfolds as a flower responding to the first spring rain.

ACTIVE RECEPTIVITY: BEING PRESENT WITH AUTHENTICITY

Subtle energy always follows thought, while soul qualities follow love. Love, in its most universal sense, is not an emotion. Love is a state of being infused with a deep awareness of the interconnection of all-that-is. We recognize the truth that we are one and all barriers dissolve. It is not a movement of action: love is a stance of just being there. Loving ourselves is in fact the movement of loving others. As we stand as witness for the other in an environment of love we see all there is, strengths, qualities, and weaknesses alike. As we stay in touch with what comes up, we identify the beauty of all that is without judgment. We radiate compassion. Bearing witness to something and staying with it is the process of transpersonal caring. Whenever there is love, there is healing and transformation (Schoch, 2005).

Active Receptivity: A nurse-healer in the postmodern world creates an atmosphere of openness and safety, which invites compassion, clarity, and truth to enter. To effectively do this, the nurse must radiate her or his own soul qualities. A nonjudging presence invites those same qualities, which are innately present in the soul of all human beings, to flow from the other. This creates a shared environment that potentiates the self-healing capacity of both the person and the nurse.

The essence of being is the energy body of the soul, which, although it cannot be observed, can be felt as an atmosphere much as the climactic conditions of the earth (Fisher, 1996, pp. 93–103). The *physical aura* is a vibration of body cells that creates an electrical-chemical movement that forms a light aura around the body, radiating the essence of the body. The movement of brain cells create brain waves and the *mental aura,* radiating the essence of thought. And, finally, we emit a *quality aura* through out-of-body consciousness, which is anchored in the invisible heart chakra over its physical center. It emanates from our soul, radiating as the essence of being. This magnetic field environment radiating from our outer heart chakra reflects our spiritual ego just as the personality is a reflection of our mind ego.

The centers for the essence of the divine, our spiritual ego, are located in the abstract world, the home of the soul.

- The divine spark, our core *self*, is a direct extension of the Source and is our unique spark of life. It is the highest vibrational energy spectrum of humankind. At this level we experience oneness with all-that-is.
- The spiritual ego creates the region of the abstract world comprised of three levels:
  - Will—the intent behind the creative impulse. When put forward with resolve—will power—it calls forth a germinal idea and begins the process of movement towards form.
  - Wisdom—pure focused attention that links our intuition or inner wisdom to primordial intelligence; the quintessence of all our previous life experiences housed in the spiritual ego. People with adequately developed mental clairvoyance can read the Akasic Records, the universal record of all events across time housed in the etheric field.
  - Active intelligence—the upper sphere of the thought world, which serves as the gateway into the abstract world. When contacted through simple awareness, an intuitive shift in the focal point from the concrete to our abstract world occurs. An opening and outpouring of the soul also occurs simultaneously.
- The soul holds the seed crystal of our destiny and life purpose, along with the unique potential that is available to us throughout our life. It is also home of the universal spiritual qualities such as love and compassion, joy and peace, which reside in the soul of all human beings. It is located in the energy vortex, situated in the sixth dimension over our heart chakra. Intuition, housed in the soul, is often referred to as our inner wisdom, because at this level we experience our true intelligence and our conscience. We access a knowing that transcends our own, and integrate it with the wisdom of our body-mind to create a holistic perspective.
- Our spiritual ego facilitates a sense of balance and harmony, enhancing our energy as we naturally synchronize the frequencies of our core self with the rhythms of the universe. From a centered position we see clearly the reality in front of us. We can sense into ourselves and into others, identifying common themes and areas of misalignment.

When we approach life from the perspective of the abstract world, our vibrational energy rises to a threshold that activates our universal spiritual qualities, creating an environment of harmlessness. This generates a sense of trustworthiness and unconditional regard, which enhances the energy field of those around us (Price, 1997, pp. 51–59).

The quality aspect of the soul is the first thing that is born along with the already functioning body and brain. Qualities cannot be learned, they simply are, as manifest in babies and small children. They neither come from the past nor move into the future, so we cannot identify with them. All we can do is simply be in touch with them. And this requires surfing between the regions of concrete and abstract thought, which is initiated through the expression of "slow feelings."

Emotions are always present at the body-mind level, playing a very important part in human evolution. Before joy there was fear; without fear there can be no survival. Brain research has demonstrated that "fast feelings" of fear and aggression belong to the reptilian and mammalian brain as part of the survival instinct (Lipton, 2005). Stimulated by emotions felt at the body level, they are reactive in nature, creating an immediate response in our concrete world. As we continue to develop associations between real and perceived threats, our body-mind cannot discern between doing and thinking about doing. This creates a hindrance not only for the manifestation of our qualities, but also for the manifestation of slow feelings, the vehicle in which the spiritual qualities are carried.

The neocortex and newly forming forebrain are home to higher mental functions; abstract thought, planning, complex memories, language, executive reasoning, logic, and the autobiographical sense of self. Slow feelings, such as inner peace, stillness, compassion, love, and joy, are not necessary for survival, but are essential to foster the continued unfolding of human potential. Entirely structured in the neocortex, forebrain, and heart energy vortex, they create out-of-body consciousness. Awareness coming from this place creates an atmosphere of nonaction, an environment of stillness.

Real power is simply the ability to create our own reality, to live our own life and fulfill our destiny. This occurs when we effectively manage both fast and slow feelings. Balance occurs when we can catch our fast feelings and shift the energy to our higher abstract world guided by slow feelings. Catching a thought creates a huge shift in perception as we experience a break with programmed response, a tiny moment of silence. Stillness is the underlying consciousness out of which every thought-form is born. Wisdom comes with the ability to be still. Being still, looking, and listening activate the nonconceptual intelligence within us, which then directs our words and actions. It fosters self-healing.

Each body-mind symptom is a manifestation of effort to get back in touch with a quality; it's the body's quest for wholeness (Schoch, 2005, p. 141). We (nurse and/or patient) must be able to witness the chaos in the illness event so that we can facilitate the reconnection process. This requires the courage of presence. To be totally present, to just observe with awareness, means we must make a relationship with the phenomenon, an act of unconditional love. Thinking and understanding limit the flow of love, while respect and unconditional regard guarantee more consciousness.

When the mind experiences the presence of total acceptance, it encounters real respite, often for the first time. Suddenly we see the truth that weaknesses are not so much the product of ourselves as they are part of being human. It is the dawning of a deep understanding that these same fears and phenomena are present in every human being in differing situations and conditions. The structure of the problem comes out of the nature of fear and the emotions it creates, a natural phenomenon, rather than a fatal personal flaw. This realization moves us closer, creating a relationship with ourselves, often for the first time. Things begin to fall into place; the journey towards wholeness has begun.

The doorway to self-healing is sadness. Sadness exists when we become aware that there is no way of doing, no way of achieving, no way of any possible action, not even through fear or anger to change the situation. Then there is only sadness. The sudden not doing creates a profound stillness; sadness is stillness. Through depersonalization, sadness is immediately transformed into stillness. When we feel self-compassion and surrender rather than self-pity and struggle, stillness will emerge. Stillness turns into a breathtaking emptiness, not devoid but filled with totality, energy not directed towards anything. This energy, full but not used, is compassion. It activates the spiritual ego, and inner wisdom guides action towards a different response. Rather than logic or control, movement flows forward on the energy of love... love in action.

Sadness is an atmosphere generated by the realization that our history has ended. Moving from fear and struggle to the acknowledgment of the hopelessness of the situation, we surrender. The moment of surrender finds us filled with a deep sadness, which, conversely, unleashes a sudden feeling of strength. It creates a deep space of stillness and awareness, generating a feeling of closeness. Surrender marks our launch on a deeply healing journey. We effortlessly begin to observe what is there. We quit asking why, we do not analyze it; we simply step outside of time into the moment. We let whatever comes up to touch us.

Nurses can help patients move from sadness, to silence, and then forward to healing. Crossing the bridge of sadness moves through several stages (Schoch, 2005, p. 155):

- learning to release—practicing forgiveness
- learning to be aware—moving into stillness
- being in relationship—connecting with things and people meaningful in our life

- having inner peace—having no need for justification
- having no reaction—reacting with slow feelings through balance
- being humble—having no need for defending; trusting in the universe

The turning point in an illness event occurs when we no longer feel a need to blame a person or event, make excuses for ourselves, or deny the truth of the situation. It is the moment of surrender. The attitude of not defending activates the soul. The less defensive we are, the more love we experience. The soul is the only thing worth protecting, and paradoxically, it is protected best by not defending. Simple, loving, and compassionate presence offers a field of total acceptance so there is no need to defend. Self-healing then begins.

BECOMING A HEALING PRESENCE

There is nothing in this world that does not involve a movement toward the soul. Nursing is a practice of serving. It has two aspects; one is to serve others, and the second, deeper meaning is the recognition that our whole being is in the service of the soul. Our presence can facilitate or hinder others in their healing efforts. Only in transpersonal relationship can each become the carrier of healing energy and love, facilitating the movement towards wholeness of both in their own unique way.

Each soul has its pattern of energy, its fundamental evolutionary movement, which means it has a clear purpose—a reason for being—which is to become what it holds within itself. Soul growth is the movement of becoming, not in the sense of knowledge or achievement, but as a blossoming into that which is dormant within us, similar to the unfolding of a flower. As our being deepens we manifest a body that can touch and be touched by others. It has looseness and a translucent quality of radiance about it. This creates an atmosphere where our innate spiritual qualities and our unique personal potential come together into a unified state of being. The wider the gap of silence between perception and thought, the more depth there is in our being, the more conscious we are. It is this rhythm between doing and being that creates the unique characteristics of one's atmosphere; it is the atmosphere of the whole that is important. Spiritual qualities include (Schoch, 2005, p. 219):

- awareness—enlarging perspective that grows out of observation and the releasing of old patterns, coupled with the process of detachment

- respect—seeing things as they are by not adding or taking away, coupled with no desire to manipulate or change them
- acknowledgment—saying yes to an observation without judgment; affirming whatever we see
- gratitude—recognizing life and its qualities, nothing more than that
- humility—refraining from power games and egoism, a stance of being, beyond engagement and struggle
- simplicity—allowing what is there to be without adding anything that does not belong; not to lie or betray or exaggerate
- trust—practicing the art of patience while not being concerned about time; trust can only come through being present in the atmosphere of qualities
- surrender—forgetting ourselves; it is faith in a process larger than ourselves
- vulnerability—allowing ourselves to be open to hurt in the psycho-spiritual sense, which creates strength
- love—moving towards what is new, which is following the flow of love

Each unique soul has a blend of characteristics that can be sensed as they are manifest in the actions and attitudes of the individual. If we live in balance between the concrete and abstract world, we walk in balance within an atmosphere of harmlessness. We are not going anywhere—not into the past or the future; there is only the moment. There is no stability either because there is only change. It is in this atmosphere that one becomes free so the soul can fly.

From this stance we learn to trust our observations without making a single compromise because of what other people say. It is our own observations, made from a heightened state of awareness, that can transform us. True presence takes courage and authenticity, which means we must stay with our observations even if they look totally wrong. Our own observations are better and closer to the/our truth. Resulting decisions and actions are in keeping with the natural flow of the situation before us.

In order to understand and express ourselves we need a certain amount of space. Providing a space for reflection and contemplation is a key requisite to healing. The less nurses are in touch with their own atmosphere, the less space they can give the patient. When we are in the presence of suffering, if we constantly try to find ways to help, it will disturb the process of the person's crossing over the bridge of sadness. As a professional caregiver, attachment to our techniques and protocols must be loose enough to allow what is new and unknown to shine through. Practices that support, rather than deny, the suffering of those we serve includes the cultivation of the still point of the heart (Tolle, 2005):

- Cultivate Stillness: To be in stillness means being in total insecurity with no reaction, no knowing, and no expectation.
- Cultivate No-Thought: Observation is the absence of thought that wants to achieve, to change, to avoid insecurity.
- Cultivate Emptiness: To be in emptiness means to be content with the "isness" of the moment. Stillness and emptiness, in movement together, become the vehicle for manifestation of our soul qualities.

A healing presence is the manifestation of unconditional acceptance. Transpersonal caring is a loving movement out of stillness, the movement towards integration of body, mind, and soul. In sharing, the unfolding of soul begins. Sharing is the ultimate movement—and only a world of sharing is truly a peaceful world.

Living from the perspective of spiritual ego versus mind ego is not something we create. There is nothing special going on. "I am awake" becomes a state of being, only experienced by an outside source. We will not be aware of how loving we are, but others will experience our love towards them. Qualities are manifest only when we are not aware of them, when we have *become* the qualities—when we *are* the atmosphere. Awareness is the absence of description; it is flow. The body-mind stops doing and thinking and becomes, instead, a carrier of energy and the qualities, much as a candle hosts the qualities of the flame. Our healing presence becomes the light for others on our shared journey towards wholeness.

Every illness is a desperate search of the body-mind to again be in relationship with its soul—to regain the ability to radiate the light of love. Consciousness is created through love; a phenomenon of "knowing" that transcends understanding. When we try to understand something intellectually we limit the movement of the vibrational energy of love which is unconditional and unlimited. The key to healing is total awareness; not just acceptance of what is in front of us, but a direct observation of whatever is present and the process that is unfolding. As the mind quits trying to judge or justify, it begins to relax and quietly observe. Events begin to effortlessly fall into place in a natural rhythm as things become simply what they are intended to be. And we move further down the healing path towards wholeness.

Manuel Schoch

BIBLIOGRAPHY

Bohm, D. (1981). The physicist and the mystic—Is a dialogue between them possible? A conversation between David Bohm and Renee Weber. *Re-Vision, 6*(1), 34–44.

Braud, W. (2000). Wellness implications of retroactive intentional influence: Exploring an outrageous hypothesis. *Alternative Therapies, 6*(1), 37–48.

Castenada, C. (1972). *Journey to Ixt.* Carlsbad, CA: Hay House.

Dossey, B., Keegan, L., Guzetta, C. R., & Kolkmeier, L. G. (1995). *Holistic nursing: A handbook for practice* (2nd Ed.) Gaithersberg, MD: Aspen.

Dwyer, W. W. (2004). *The power of intention: Learning to co-create your world your way.* Carlsbad, CA: Hay House.

Fisher, B. (1996). *Man-grand reflection of the greater cosmos: Studies in occult anatomy.* (Vol. 3.) Prescott, AZ: Subru.

Kurtz, E., & Ketcham, K. (1992). *The spirituality of imperfection: Storytelling and the search for meaning.* New York: Bantam.

Kuthumi, D. K. (1996). *The human aura: How to activate and energize your aura and chakras.* Corwin Springs, MT. Summit University Press.

Lipton, B. (2005). *The biology of belief: Unleashing the power of consciousness, matter and miracles.* Santa Rosa, CA: Mountain Love.

Madrid, M., & Barrett, E.A.M. (Eds.). (1994). *Roger's scientific art of nursing practice.* New York: National League for Nursing Press.

Newman, M. (1986). *Health as expanding consciousness.* St. Louis, MO: C. V. Mosby.

Parse, R. R. (1995). *Illuminations: The human becoming theory in practice and research.* New York: National League for Nursing Press.

Pesut, D., & Hermann, J. (1999). *Clinical reasoning: The art and science of critical and creative thinking.* Boston: Delmar.

Price, J. R. (1997). *A spiritual philosophy for the new world.* Carlsbad, CA: Hay House.

Schoch, M. (2005). *Healing with qualities: The essence of time therapy.* Boulder, CO: Sentient.

Tolle, E. (1999). *The power of now: A guide to spiritual enlightenment.* Novato, CA: New World Library.

Tolle, E. (2003). *Stillness speaks.* Novato, CA: New World Library.

Tolle, E. (2005). *A new earth: awakening to your life's purpose.* New York: Penguin.

Watson, J. (1999). *Postmodern nursing and beyond.* New York: Churchill Livingston.

Woody, C. (2004). *Standing stark: Willingness to engage.* Prescott, AZ: Kenosis.

SECTION IV

A Healing Path: Weaving a Purposeful Life

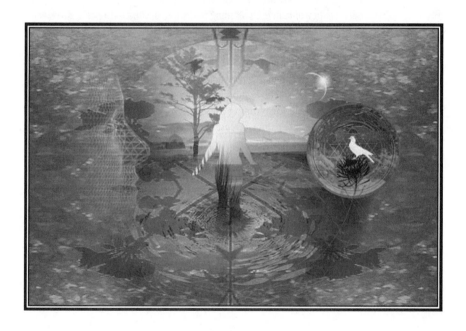

Life is a celebratory event.
Let us choose the forces of
life which will safeguard
the beauty of life.
Through hope, vision,
courage and will,
we create a purposeful life which
celebrates itself.

Upanishads

CHAPTER 8

Authentic Living
The Path of Becoming

It takes courage to grow up and turn out to be who you really are.

e. e. cummings

Our being, the very essence of our life, is in a constant state of change. We are tangible. Unique. Present. Embodied. Evolving. And we are witnessing a great mystery: the discovery of the self-organizing, self-synthesizing, and infinitely creative process moving through the cosmos—and ourselves. As we truly grasp the power of the ever-unfolding and evolving Spirit of the Universe, we realize that we are on sacred ground. While we recognize that we are in charge of our individual destiny, we often forget that we are also part of a larger, eternal human and universal destiny. In reality, we are not separate from each other, from nature, or from spirit. Universal Spirit connects the inner and outer being of all in a continuous and ever-changing dance of life.

Nursing is a profession called into being by the society it serves. We come to our work with a noble purpose: the aspiration for service. Supporting others facing a health challenge or a life passage such as birth and death requires us to take ourselves out of the center and put spirit in our place. While we cannot fully understand or describe spirit, Fetzer Institute has crafted a description intended not to be definitive, but rather to be framing for shared consideration:

> By spirit we mean the Universal Spirit that is the deepest and most inclusive ground of being. Spirit is the source of all that exists. Spirit is the infinite, creative energy that gives birth to the universe. Spirit is the common source of the world's faith traditions. Spirit is the love that creates and sustains life. (Lehman, 2004, pp. 11–13)

It is the spiritual values of compassion and caring that unite our nursing mission and identity. Healing and wholeness emerge from the spirit orientation of our service. Together we draw upon the scientific, educational, and religious/philosophical resources that free the powers of love, forgiveness, and healing that reside in every human being.

The field and object perspective of wholeness observes life as a complimentary dance of being and doing, a path of choicelessness and also of choice. We like to choose because we enjoy being in control. Paradoxically, we make choices within the context of a choiceless existence. We did not choose our parents, our culture, or our language, at least consciously. However, we did choose our profession, our significant relationships, and the manner in which we approach life. Total emphasis on choice leads to anxiety, while adherence to choicelessness leads to passivity. It is the appropriate mix and movement between our acceptance of choicelessness and the dynamism of choice that creates the most vibrant dance of life.

Choiceless things must be accepted unconditionally in order to bring harmony to our lives. We are human beings, which calls us to an unconditional acceptance of the human family. We are also made of spirit and unconditional love, so it is not an optional extra. Love is choiceless, but the ways we choose to express it are optional. Choicelessness is not fatalism; it is not passive. It is an active acceptance of reality—an "isness." It is getting into alignment with our being; our vocation, our destiny. From that context we make choices through the expression of our creativity, imagination, and improvisational capacity (Kumar, 2004, pp. 32–35).

The unity of life manifests in millions of forms, but each form makes our own particular contribution to the movement of the whole. We are born with our own unique gifts, the essence of our natural self. The complimentarity of being and doing flows out of our authentic self. Therefore, choices that are not made out of our true identity will inevitably lead us astray.

Nurses who walk in balance are in touch with their authenticity. A balanced life is a life of acceptance and alignment. They receive whatever is given to them from the process of the universe and the natural order as a gift. Received with gratitude and joy rather than struggle and resistance, they flow in harmony with the natural order. From that context conscious choices are made regarding the particulars that enhance their life journey in a manner that fulfills the destiny of their soul.

EXPANDING CONSCIOUSNESS: A SHIFT IN VALUES

Values are a reflection of consciousness. They are the driving force and motivation for the choices and actions that guide our life. Ethical behavior is of necessity conscious behavior. *Values are developmental in nature.* As persons mature, their worldview and set of values enlarge. Increasing awareness expands their circle of relationships, bringing a greater sense of autonomy, accountability, and authenticity as they actualize their potential more fully (Hall, 1986).

Developmental theorists have identified specific stages of development from infancy throughout adulthood. In nested hierarchy, each stage has specific tasks to be accomplished that prepare us for the next phase. Once we have completed all seven stages the cycle repeats at higher levels of complexity, refining our capacity as we now have a full range of basic values to draw from in each situation encountered. See Figure 8.1. The values stages include the following:

- Stage One: Safety: Physical and Psychological
  - Values such as: security, health, order, fairness, trust
- Stage Two: Relationships: Self and other
  - Values such as: open communication, courtesy, respect, conflict resolution
- Stage Three: Self-esteem: Skills and power
  - Values such as: competence, boundaries, emotional intelligence, balance
- Stage Four: Transformation: Doing and being
  - Values such as: creativity, teamwork, flexibility, logic

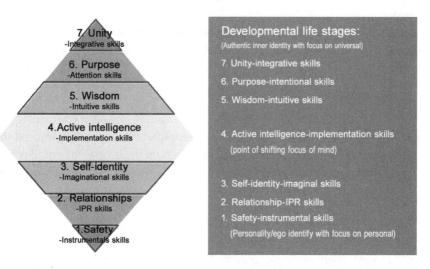

FIGURE 8.1   Seven stages of conscious leadership model (values, developmental stages, and skill sets).

- Stage Five: Intuition: Pattern recognition
  - Values such as: wisdom, cooperation, adaptability, meaning
- Stage Six: Intent: Purpose and goals
  - Values such as: service, generosity, insight, patience
- Stage Seven: Unity: Balanced wholeness
  - Values such as: contemplation, forgiveness, humility, ethics

Our journey is a continuous dance between doing and being—the evolution of spirit ever moving forward. The first three stages of values focus on our capacity for doing, while the final three encompass our capacity for being. A solid foundation creates a framework for higher dimensional values that offer healing to the world. We increase ability in surfing between the two worlds by expanding our transformational values.

It is the human condition to reach beyond the comfort of the known and familiar, it is our destiny. Each step we take is an open choice. *Choices are based upon, and reflect, our core values.* Choice is a matter of judgment, a dangerous sword. On one hand, perennial wisdom guides us not to judge, while in day-to-day decisions we must make judgments. Each decision has consequences that will either secure the status quo, create a new roadmap, or transform old ways that defy our rational understanding. When we withdraw from open-minded inquiry and expansive choices, new possibilities fall away as we are held captive by interests other than the truth. Life calls us daily to make values-based choices in response to the movements of spirit. What we focus on and how we choose to answer that call makes all the difference.

Nested in the juncture between past and future, a choice point always occurs in the moment; the now. A choice point is a moment of truth where we have to decide our next steps. Choices are strongly influenced by our point of focus, guided by a cluster of values that are a mirror of our consciousness:

- *Choice based on the first three levels of value are primarily externally referenced.* When we are in the first three levels of development, we tend to rely on the rules of family, the wisdom from the experts in clinical practice, and lessons that worked in the past. We are testing the foundation built by others, discerning what is and is not "my truth."

If we approach a choice point with a fragile identity, we focus on "can I do this?" If our past is filled with a sense of failure or inadequacy we will experience anxiety about moving forward. Our decisions will be incremental and controlling. If the future is not compelling, if we do not have an inspiring

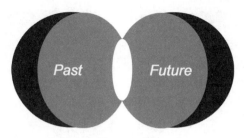

Reliable self
Issues based

FIGURE 8.2   Dynamics of doing.

vision of what might be, we will find a significant change daunting for the small gain seen. See Figure 8.2.

Healing wounds of the past or being inspired by a powerful futuristic vision are two ways to encourage a choice that has the potential to further our development and our capacities, rather than selecting the status quo. Partnering a novice with an expert is another way to encourage risk-taking behavior leading to enhanced skill and mastery.

- *Choices based on higher-level values are internally referenced.* As our capacity and awareness grows, our value stage shifts from a focus of doing to higher stages of being. As we become clear about who we are and what we are about, the most powerful influence on choice is our higher-stage values. At core, it is these values that guide ethical decisions in complex situations. As we mature and evolve, when we feel stuck or undecided, it is not usually because we do not have enough information; rather, it is because there is a conflict between our values and what the situation is asking from us. See Figure 8.3.

We begin to become more authentic and transparent in our decision making. We start to bring creativity, flexibility, and playfulness to the moment. We increasingly test the requests and viewpoints of others; take broader risks, and collaborate in a cocreative fashion. We begin to share our viewpoints with others, becoming part of the evidence-based practice that others refer to as they begin their own professional journey.

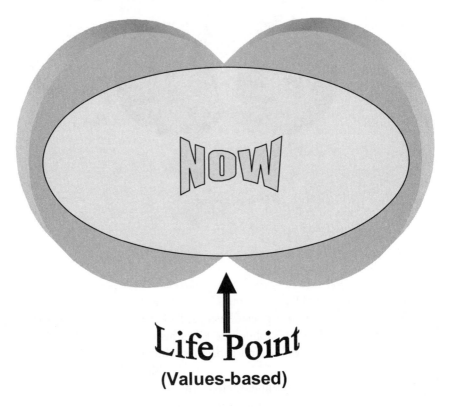

FIGURE 8.3   Dynamics of being.

A BALANCED VALUES MATRIX: INTEGRATING THE PERSONAL AND PROFESSIONAL

The complexities of the twenty-first-century health care system demand dynamic and vibrant nurses who provide service and compassion to the public. The one essential quality of today's professionals is that they must be their own person, authentic in every regard.

Nurses are professional knowledge workers whose wisdom falls into several domains:

- Nursing Science: knowledge for understanding
  - Ability to understand scientific laws and principles
  - Ability to analyze and evaluate

- • Ability to bring logic and reason to decision making
- • Ability to make judgments and conclusions from relevant data
- • Nursing Art: knowledge for clinical care and safety
  - • Ability to analyze the current situation from multiple perspectives
  - • Ability to recognize and comprehend the subtle patterns underlying the phenomenon being viewed
  - • Ability to join and integrate seemingly unrelated parts into a larger whole
  - • Ability to synthesize findings into creation of new order
- • Nursing Presence: knowledge for quality and creation of meaning
  - • Ability to establish meaningful connections
  - • Ability to grasp significance and meaning unfolding for the client
  - • Ability to witness without interference in client's process
  - • Ability to conduct oneself in a moral manner

A knowledge professional whose style is consistent with his or her personality and character is autonomous, highly independent, practices with solid values, develops enduring relationships, and leads from the heart. Such a nurse demonstrates self-discipline, identifies his or her own growth edge, and continues to develop skills and capacities while integrating them into a unified whole.

Values development continues across the life span and, for nurses, can be categorized into two dimensions: personal and professional. The predominant value clusters between the two worlds create a specific pattern of self-management, which fosters an explicit leadership style in personal and organizational life:

- • *Personal Values:* Those values that guide and shape our inner landscape of beliefs and aspirations that satisfy our basic needs for connection and meaning.
- • *Professional Values:* Those values that guide and shape our external world of work and society that satisfy our basic needs for contribution and community.
- • *Leadership Style:* The unique clustering of values in both the personal and professional domains, giving rise to a certain pattern of self-management and leadership that is manifest in our private and organizational life.

Based on the developmental work of Barrett (1998), Maslow (1980), Erikson (1980), Benner (1984), Drucker (1999), and Rogers (1980), the values

Personal Values Stage	Professional Values Stage	Leadership Style
Self Actualization-Wholeness	Older-Completion Focus	Prophetic-Universal Style
Intention-Purpose & Goals	Maturing-Contribution Focus	Servant-Partner Style
Intuition-Inner Wisdom	Reflective-Collaboration Focus	Collaborative-Democratic Style
Shifting Focus-Active Intelligence	Growing-Independence Focus	Facilitating-Enabling Style
Self Esteem-Skill & Power	Young-Identity Focus	Bureaucratic-Institutional Style
Relationships-Love & Belonging	Beginning-Fitting In Focus	Paternal-Relational Style
Safety-Physical & Psychological	Launching-Skill Focus	Authoritarian-Controlling Style

FIGURE 8.4   Leadership style reflects values.

and associated stages of personal, professional, and leadership progression were mapped into the matrix found in Figure 8.4. Balance, self-empowerment, and authenticity are the outcome when integration of these dynamic principles occurs.

SEVEN STAGES OF PERSONAL DEVELOPMENT: LIVING FROM A FOUNDATION OF BALANCE

The most profound gift we can offer ourselves, our loved ones, and the world at large is to be a happy, whole, and balanced being. Authentic people are dedicated to developing a strong foundation so they can live and walk in balance. When all aspects of us are in balance, we are centered, vibrant, and filled with a sense of well-being.

The context for our life and our body-mind-spirit system is divided into seven centers that reflect the seven bodies of consciousness that comprise the human being. At various periods in our life our values cluster into certain stages/centers with choices and decisions primarily made from that level of consciousness (Choquette, 2000):

- Solid Foundation: Confident survival instincts with safe home base
- Strength and Vitality: Creative expression and healthy emotional connections
- Skill and Power: Self-esteem guided by ability, motivation, and personal power
- Integration: Relationships flowing from both personal and spiritual connections
- Expression: Authentic communication with intuition and integrity

- Intent: Conscious awareness and clear life vision
- Wholeness: Capacity to connect to all things and the universal

A well-developed and balanced body moves with strength, vibrancy, and grace. Personal growth is a developmental process that follows a predictable pattern and a hierarchy of needs. As our needs are met and we become aligned with our life purpose, we feel physically grounded, emotionally safe, mentally clear, centered in giving and receiving love, creative and effective in self-expression, inspired and intentional in choosing, and intimately connected to and guided by the universe. This natural state for human existence leads to a satisfying, productive, and fulfilling life that is filled with vitality, love, creativity, blessings, and grace.

Center 1: Solid Foundation: meeting our basic needs for survival and having what is required to feel confident in the world.

Values: Survival/Safety

Characteristics of this stage:

Starting Point	Balanced
Insecure and anxious	Confident and calm
Vulnerable and threatened	Secure and safe
Scarcity mentality	Abundance mentality
Isolated and self-conscious	Connected and self-reliant
Aggressive and manipulative	Disciplined and trustworthy

This perspective creates the necessary foundation for life and living. When we feel threatened our focus shifts to this level, and decisions are made in favor of tactics that assure survival.

Center 2: Strength and Vitality: experiencing the joy of being alive in full relationship to life through sensual and emotional fulfillment as well as creative expression.

Values: Relationships / Belonging

Characteristics of this stage:

Starting Point	Balanced
Avoids or controls feelings	Embraces and honors feelings
Lives in head	Lives in whole body
Self-denies and self-neglects	Spontaneous and self-nurturing

| Focus on work & productivity | Focuses on life & self-expression |
| Lives in isolation | Lives in relationship |

This perspective activates all senses, providing sexual and creative energy as well as instinctual and emotional feelings. When we feel isolated or alone our focus shifts to this level, and decisions are made in favor of tactics that assure inclusion.

Center 3: Self-Esteem: experiencing self-direction, physical energy, and personal expression of power.

Values: Self Esteem/Autonomy

Characteristics of this stage:

Starting Point	Balanced
Defensive & harsh	Patient & gentle
Weak & timid	Powerful & strong
Directs & suspects	Listens & trusts
Workaholic overachiever	Balanced confidence
Victim mode	Partnership mode

This perspective serves as a gateway for emotions and anger. Intellectually it influences our decision making and personal power, while emotionally it guides our ability to trust our intuition and instincts. When we feel inadequate our focus shifts to this level and we make decisions in favor of self-promotion and control.

Center 4: Integration: experiencing balance in emotions and actions by connecting the body-mind with higher spiritual wisdom.

Values: Transformation / Mastery

Characteristics of this stage:

Starting Point	Balanced
Exclusive of others	Inclusive with others
Superior to others	Part of the human family
Righteous & judging	Compassionate & humble
Experiences ethnic divisions	Sees equality in diversity
Consistent struggle	Flow & synchronicity

Of special note to healers: Another person's vital energy (nonlocally) often hits us at the heart chakra, especially when we are sympathetic. Empathy allows us to witness others' suffering without taking it into our energy system.

Empathy training for professionals includes the following competencies:

1. Know yourself: learning to identify and feel your own emotions
2. Practice emotional management: controlling your emotions in the motivation and service of your own goals
3. Practice empathy: experiencing the emotions of others without identifying with them by maintaining your objectivity
4. Manage emotional relationships: developing and maintaining good intrapersonal and interpersonal relationships over time

This perspective is the point of transformation, connecting the lower body/mind with higher soul/wisdom. It serves as the center for balance for the entire body-mind-spirit, fostering altruism, compassion, forgiveness, understanding, and love. When we feel superior we are stuck at this level, making decisions in favor of an agenda that is exclusively focused on our ideas and intent.

Center 5: Authentic Expression: experiencing communication with integrity directly from your inner voice—intuition, thoughts, beliefs, and ideas—as you introduce your spirit to the world.

Values: Intuition/Knowing

Characteristics of this stage:

Starting Point	Balanced
Muddled mind chatter	Intuitive knowing
Drone of confusion	Focused clarity
Influenced by mass consciousness	Influenced by instincts
Taking things at face value	Seeing the deeper meaning
Guided by thinking and planning	Guided by inner knowing

This perspective serves as the center of expression and creativity, as well as our ability to connect with the expression of others—laying the foundation for understanding. When we feel confusion we focus on this level, making decisions that minimize risk.

Center 6: Clear Intent: experiencing your personal life vision with its purpose and goals clearly seen and understood.

Values: Intent/Purpose

Characteristics of this stage:

Starting Point	Balanced
Emphasizes appearance	Honest in self expression
Difficulty conveying ideas to others	Expresses self with clarity
Delusions or overexpectations	Accurate view of situation
Controlling perfectionist	Accepting of all perspectives
Over-intellectualizing	Balanced understanding

This perspective enhances quality of thought and all aspects of mind, including intuitive wisdom. When we feel misunderstood we focus on this level, making observations and promises that are unrealistic and off center.

Center 7: Balanced Wholeness: experiencing your highest wisdom and personal expression while bringing light to the world.

Values: Ethics/Spirituality

Characteristics of this stage:

Starting Point	Balanced
Sees things in isolation	Sees all as interconnected
Restless and uncertain	Calm and centered
Confused about deep issues	Clear self-knowing
Hyperactive and outspoken	Gentle and compassionate
Anxious and concerned	Tranquil and peaceful

This perspective serves as the center for our highest spiritual consciousness and personal expression, connecting us to the source of Life. When we experience deep anxiety over a large family/social issue we focus on this level, which fosters a need to convert others to our perspective.

Values Matrix—The I-MAP

Models are tools that represent and describe things that are intangible and invisible. An I-MAP Model depicts individual values, creating a pattern that models their level of consciousness. See Figure 8.5.

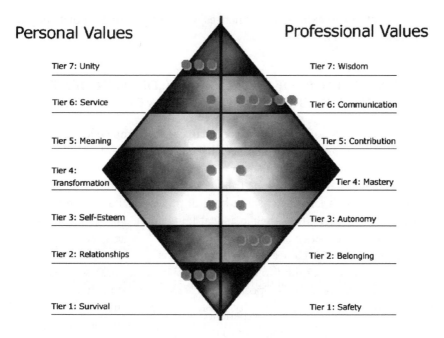

Personal Values   Professional Values

Tier 7: Unity   Tier 7: Wisdom

Tier 6: Service   Tier 6: Communication

Tier 5: Meaning   Tier 5: Contribution

Tier 4: Transformation   Tier 4: Mastery

Tier 3: Self-Esteem   Tier 3: Autonomy

Tier 2: Relationships   Tier 2: Belonging

Tier 1: Survival   Tier 1: Safety

FIGURE 8.5   Personal and professional values matrix.

The values that comprise these seven centers are initially developed during the first phase of life, with modification and refinement occurring across the life span (Lewis, 1991):

- *Values Stages:* A clustering of related values reflects a stage of development with defining characteristics regarding overall level of conscious awareness. The next stage can be attained by establishing and pursuing growth strategies for further maturation and development, if our life experiences are embraced and reviewed for the learning that they offer.
- *Values Gap:* Occasionally a level of personal or professional development has no identified values. When the gap is in only one dimension of our life, it may be something unconsciously taken care of or it points to the next stage of growth. If the gap is consistent in both the personal and professional domain, it may indicate an unfinished developmental task that could be revisited and completed.

A healthy individual moves easily from one level to the other, as life circumstance demands. However, if we have not developed the core capacities in a specific area, we are destined to go back to complete that developmental task, or continue to experience challenges when we get stuck in that specific area (Izzo & Withers, 1996).

SEVEN STAGES OF PROFESSIONAL DEVELOPMENT: PRACTICING FROM THE PERSPECTIVE OF MASTERY

Professional mastery encompasses more than clinical competence: it includes a moral, ethical, and caring presence that performs the role of nurse in a comprehensive and inclusive manner (Leonard, 1992). Mastery is not perfection, but rather a journey, and the true master must be willing to try and fail and try again. To a large extent, the kind of professional a person becomes depends on the strength of their personal foundation. The professional self emerges from the personal through values, intent, beliefs, and goals that inform and guide their clinical choices and actions.

The development of the professional self follows the same sequence that the personal self experiences. Specific tasks achieved in sequential order lead to the evolving sense of authenticity, mastery, and wholeness. Research suggests that it takes approximately 3 years to develop mastery of basic nursing practice, and then the nurse becomes a guide for others (Benner, 1984; Benner, Tanner, & Chesla, 1996).

The following seven stages of professional development have been identified as essential for a healthy and vibrant professional practice (Erikson, 1980; Leddy & Pepper, 1989):

- Launching professional   Focus on skill
- Beginning professional   Focus on fit
- Young professional   Focus on identity
- Growing professional   Focus on independence
- Reflective professional   Focus on collaboration
- Maturing professional   Focus on contribution
- Older professional   Focus on completion

The quality of goal achievement in one stage will strongly influence movement to the next level. Successful completion of each stage greatly influences later role achievement. While it is important to focus on clinical skill competency (especially in the first three stages of professional development), equally important are other aspects of role development. It is process-oriented skills such as communicating, evaluating, educating, collaborating, and advocating that guide and enlarge clinical understanding and engagement with the patient and others on the health team. Expanding competency in inquiry and experimentation, comfort with ambiguity, clarity in communication as well as decisive and moral action, is the hallmark of a reflective practitioner (Mezirow et al., 1991).

Stage 1: Launching professional—Focus on skill

Values: Survival/Safety

The goals of a new nurse entering practice are: to develop trust in one's preceptors and managers, to effectively develop their abilities to fulfill professional role requirements, to be able to count on others to assist them in meeting patient objectives, to experience gratification in their new role, and to receive recognition for a job well done.

Characteristics of this stage:

Productive:

- Trust in self and team members with strong sense of accomplishment
- Energy focused on meeting client needs
- Optimism regarding professional development across career and commitment to lifelong learning

Nonproductive:

- Mistrusts self and professional peers with guarded relationships
- Doubts own competency with energy focused on meeting own needs
- Focus on short-term tasks versus long-range goals

Stage 2: Beginning professional—Focus on fit

Values: Relationships/Belonging

After successful initiation into the profession, the goals expand: to depend on more mature professionals for guidance some of the time, to experience self as a professional in one's own right, to know that others on the team value one's presence and contribution, to admit that "not knowing so let's find out" is a sign of strength rather than weakness.

Characteristics of this stage:

Productive:

- Trusts self as competent and knowledgeable
- Trusts clients' wisdom regarding their own care
- Develops effective interpersonal relationships that demonstrate collaboration

Nonproductive:

- Views self as servant who carries out orders given by others
- Views self and client as subordinates versus partners in the health care team
- Maintains procedural focus

Stage 3: Young professional—Focus on identity

Values: Self-Esteem /Autonomy

The young professional now experiences a deeper sense of competency in the role, seeks experiences to independently expand his or her knowledge in a specific area of practice, seeks a mentor to learn the wisdom of a master rather than textbook learning. A nurse at this stage is ideal as a preceptor to RNs new to the field, or those returning after an extended period away from the practice. Participation in unit-based projects facilitates organizational skill development at this stage.

Characteristics of this stage:

Productive:

- Offers creative ideas for development of alternatives in problem solving
- Takes risks in carrying out advocacy role for client, accepting account-ability for decisions and actions
- Begins to share new found wisdom through preceptor role with new graduates and young professionals

Nonproductive:

- Relies on policy rather than taking initiative
- Seeks reward for efficiency versus sound judgment and is more com-fortable with routine than independent decisions
- Accountable to employer rather than client

Stage 4: Growing professional—Focus on independence

Values: Transformation/Mastery

Professional identity is enlarging along with a personal belief system about the discipline of nursing; skill in area of specialty practice expands; compe-tency in experimentation is leading to an expanding awareness of the nursing role in implementing planned change through partnerships and teamwork. A nurse at this stage of development serves in an expanding clinical practice role, as a charge nurse, or as a preceptor to experienced nurses returning to school.

Characteristics of this stage:

Productive:

- Expansion of professional network to increase competency
- Behavior promoting initiative rather than conformity
- Seeks continuing education to further develop role rather than out of a sense of duty

Nonproductive:

- Feels inadequate rather than professionally competent
- Feels other-directed rather than self-directed
- Feels others control practice; has no time for professional tasks as assigned procedural tasks consume all the time available

Stage 5: Reflective professional—Focus on collaboration

Values: Intuition/Knowing

Professional identity now expands from independence to interdependence with clients, peers, and other colleagues in the health care delivery system; mutual assessment of total needs of client, family and community; awareness and respect for the unique contributions of each discipline, determining who is best qualified for the aspect of care required; evaluation of the health care system including policy and reward structures. Beginning leadership positions as well as mentor roles with other experienced professionals occurs at this level of development.

Characteristics of this stage:

Productive:

- Values clinical practice and serves as a mentor to other nurses
- Values discovery and learning, continuously engaged as a consumer of research findings, and contributes to the literature
- Positively impacts society's image of nursing through role modeling behavior

Nonproductive:

- Leaves client with experience of nursing as attendant and mechanical rather than professional and dynamic
- Creates a public image of nursing as technical with restorative care as only focus
- Leaves profession feeling burned out and unfulfilled, having missed multiple opportunities within the profession

Stage 6: Maturing professional—Focus on contribution values

Values: Intent/Purpose

The maturing professional develops goals for others in nursing, contributing to society through efforts in nursing education, practice, and research; experiences the value of practice with clients while mentoring or leading nursing groups; values nursing education by teaching future professionals as well as consuming and contributing to nursing literature; conducts research that substantiates significance of nursing while also acting as consumer of nursing research. Society's image of professional nursing is largely influenced by this level of professional development.

Characteristics of this stage:

Productive:

- Emergence of effective collegial, collaborative, and interpersonal relationships with clients/families/colleagues/coworkers/community
- Mutual interdisciplinary collaboration and role delegation with client as active partner
- Unique contributions to the nursing discipline through organizational leadership, publication of new knowledge gained through professional activities, and regional-national contribution

Nonproductive:

- Competition for the benefit of self versus the vulnerable client
- Practices in isolation due to lack of collaborative skills and insight into others' roles, minimizing impact of care for client
- Health care team experiences nurse as inflexible and dehumanizing

Stage 7: Older professional—Focus on completion

Values: Unity/Wholeness

The older professional has opportunities and obligations to complete unfinished business while reflecting on and cherishing their significant contributions and relationships; to offer support and strongly influence the future of nursing through interaction with young professionals, associations, and organizations that would benefit from their integrity and their longitudinal perspective on the field.

Characteristics of this stage:

Productive:

- Great personal satisfaction regarding contribution made to the profession and the people served through the years

- Passing on of dreams and accomplishments to younger professionals and society
- Pleasure in the achievement of those who follow them

Nonproductive:

- Professional identity marked by a sense of despair
- Cannot recount accomplishments of self or others to celebrate contributions made
- Feels alienated, unsupported, and alone

Personal/Professional Development Exemplar

Utilizing the values profiling tool developed in conjunction with the American Association of Critical Care Nurses and the American Home Health Association, the values profiles and weighted values cluster found in Figure 8.6 were obtained (Bodensteiner, 2001).

The values profile of the two following nurses is reflective of their level of professional development and their experiences in the world:

- Nurse 1 is a 21-year-old female with an ADN in Nursing, who is in the sixth month of her first career experience. Her Values Profile shows major focus on activities surrounding building a solid foundation in both personal and professional aspects of her life. Her values clustered at a Stage 3 level of development.

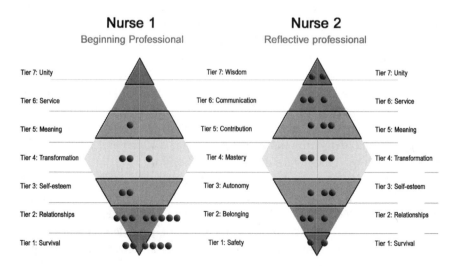

FIGURE 8.6   Professional nurse profiles.

- Nurse 2 is a 54-year-old female with a diploma in nursing, who is in the 32nd year of her career. Her Values Profile shows a well-balanced profile in both the personal and professional domains, with values clustering at Stage 5.

Each profile is an exquisite picture of a life-in-progress. It is a graphic depiction of the various stages of development we master during a meaningful career. It also demonstrates the dynamic possibilities for a continuing evolution towards mastery when we engage deeply with life.

SEVEN STAGES OF SELF-MANAGEMENT AND LEADERSHIP: LEADING FROM THE POWER OF AUTHENTICITY

Postmodern society is witnessing the emergence of the knowledge worker; a highly skilled and autonomous creative person whose intelligence is replacing the tools and machines of the industrial age.

> The most valuable assets of the 20th century were its equipment and its laborers. The most valuable asset of a 21st century institution, whether business or service industry, will be its knowledge workers and their productivity. (Drucker, 1999, p. 2)

In this new information age, knowledge workers such as nurses define their own contributions and innovations, depending on the situation. They are responsible for their own information management and communication. They alone must create and manage relationships that further their work. A knowledge worker is continuously learning, as well as teaching and mentoring. And it is this individual who is responsible for the quality experience of the person served. This requires each knowledge worker to become a self-empowered leader in ever-enlarging circles of influence.

Real power is the capacity to shift the focal point between concrete and abstract thought in such a way that self-management defines our life, rather than passively responding to it. Therefore, everyone is a manager in some sphere of their world. In the new era of the knowledge worker, rather than a formal title, a leader is any individual who holds a vision and courageously pursues it in a way that invites others to join the effort.

Development across the life span moves us to increasingly discover our potential and become more fully who we are. Knowledge is power, and consequently, knowledge of ourselves provides self-empowerment; the guiding force for the actions we take in life. Authentic leaders are dedicated to developing themselves because they know that becoming an active agent of change, rather than a passive reactor, is a lifelong process.

Our level of conscious awareness and personal power defines our leadership capacity. Leadership emerges out of the ability to link our external capacity for action (organizational and political positions, titles, educational degrees, material possessions) to our internal worldview (values, beliefs, intentions, and life purpose). A specific leadership style will foster characteristic behaviors among the group of followers. It is important to remember that any leadership style can be appropriate or inappropriate for the tasks of the organization depending on the situation (Barrett, 1998).

Leadership capacity is developmental; as our skills and awareness increase, values shift and the range of styles available to us increase, offering more flexibility and hardiness in our leadership role. The seven styles of leadership include:

- Authoritarian manager: the controlling stage
- Paternal manager: the relational stage
- Bureaucratic manager: the institutional stage
- Collaborative manager/leader: the enabling stage
- Authentic leader: the democratic stage
- Servant leader: the partner stage
- Prophetic leader: the universal stage

The movement towards accountability is a lifelong developmental process. Each stage of growth moves us further from our originating self-centered focus on survival and control towards a self-aware capacity for leadership through service. Our actions increasingly move from the innocence and ignorance of childhood towards the conscious choice and clear intent of an accountable adult. The catalyst for this dynamic growth is experiential learning supported by the presence of a mentor or leader who has completed the tasks we are striving to accomplish. It is important to note that a leadership style generates and often is supported by a corresponding followership style. Each stage in our development moves us increasingly into a position of supporting those who follow in a reciprocal exchange where both become more.

Style 1: Authoritarian manager: the controlling stage: moving from fear and distrust towards a beginning sense of security through basic life-skill development.

Leadership Style

- Maintains physical and social distance from others
- Makes all major decisions alone
- Seeks to control as much as possible
- Demands loyalty to her/him as well as the unit/organization

Follower Behaviors

- Views the leader as distant and unapproachable
- Follows passively with blind obedience
- Sees the leader as having an aura of infallibility around him/her
- Demonstrates infantile-type behavior

Characteristics of this stage:

Starting Point	Well-Developed
Insecure and dependent	Secure and dependent
Isolated	Becoming connected
Uninformed	Seeking information
Helpless and hopeless	Helpful and hopeful

Impact of style on group/organization:

This style may be necessary in times of imminent danger. However, it becomes destructive when the environment is secure. Such a leader has difficulty delegating any activities that may diminish their power. This style is particularly distressful when the followers hold values on a more advanced level, experiencing the leader's style as oppressive and unjust.

Style 2: Paternal manager: the relational stage: moving from a parental style fostering dependency and compliance towards self-confidence with basic relational skill development.

Leadership Style

- Listens to subordinates but reserves decision making for self
- Demands loyalty to superiors
- Insures careful following of the rules

Follower Behaviors

- Feels cared for and protected
- Dependent behaviors
- Views leader as approachable but recognizes that leader has the last word

Characteristics of this stage:

Starting Point	Well-Developed
Beginning competency	Expanding skills
Stranger to the organization	Knows the culture and politics

Dependent on supervisor/leader   Supported by supervisor/leader
Other-awareness   Enlarging self-awareness

Impact of style on group/organization:

This style is appropriate when the leader is highly skilled and the followers are not, such as when a new program is being rolled out in the organization. Relationships are based on fairness and mutual respect. However, rules and protocols are expected to be followed to assure an ordered environment. This style becomes dysfunctional when excessive rigidity and perfectionism is demanded while followers are seeking more autonomy and individual responsibility.

Style 3: Bureaucratic manager: the institutional stage: moving from competition and control towards cooperation through basic collaboration/team-building skill development.

Leadership Style

- Manages by objectives with a focus on order, clear policies, and goals
- Demands respect and loyalty to the institution, its mission, and its systems
- Delegates only to those who are skilled and loyal to the institution

Follower Behaviors

- Views the leader as approachable and good listener
- Sees tasks and expected outcomes clearly through leader's articulation
- Accepts the exercise of delegated authority in defined areas

Characteristics of this stage:

Starting Point	Well-Developed
Controlling others	Increasing self-control
Self-centered ego	Increasing self-awareness
Realistic and competitive	Clear and cooperative
Skilled and striving	Expert and flowing

Impact of style on group/organization:

This level of leadership is appropriate when the leader is highly skilled in an area of specialty and followers are attempting to increase competency in this area. Skills most essential for success are interpersonal effectiveness and professional mastery. The danger of rigidity and resistance to change fosters a group-think phenomenon that limits creativity and adjust performance to meet unique needs of client. On a personal level, at this stage of leadership development a tension is beginning to form between loyalty to the institution and the desire to spend time with family and oneself.

Style 4: Collaborative manager/leader: the enabling stage: moving from a work-driven and group focus towards an organizational perspective with basic unit management skill development.

Leader Qualities

- Caught between demanding efficiency and human needs of staff
- Trying to balance institutional demands with personal values
- Highly skilled as a listener and clarifier

Follower Behaviors

- Willing to express feelings, needs, and expectations
- Spontaneously shares unique perspective in clinical situations
- Demonstrates need for good interpersonal skills

Characteristics of this stage:

Starting Point	Well-Developed
Thinking and doing	Active intelligence and being
Reactive	Reflective
Imitates boss or role model	Authentic personal style
Work with people in projects	Lead people and projects

Impact of style on group/organization:

This is a stage of confusion in the developing leader. They are less certain about their beliefs and feelings. A search for new meaning may move the person away from loyalty to the institution towards increased sensitivity to the needs of the staff and self. Decision making may be difficult due to inner conflict, fostering a time of inaction. If one gets stuck here, there is a danger of slipping back into a more bureaucratic and controlling management style.

Style 5: Authentic leader: the democratic stage: moving from career and success focus towards living one's life purpose through basic system-building skills development.

Leader Qualities

- Very democratic in leadership style
- Has clear vision about how to make institution more humane
- Able to modify rules according to personal conscience

Follower Characteristics

- Good in small group interactions
- Participates as peer in decision making with patients and colleagues
- Demonstrates need to develop collaboration skills, including conflict management

Characteristics of this Stage:

Starting Point	Well-Developed
Self-judging	Self-accepting
Anxious and pushing	Calm and allowing
Notices the obvious	True visionary
Tentative about life	Confident of life purpose

Impact of style on group/organization:

This leadership style is ideal for managing a professional group of knowledge workers. Passing through the last stage, the leader now has a new sense of personal creative energy and clear vision for the work of the organization. Because of the high level of interaction among staff, support structures must be established to facilitate sharing of ideas and problems in real time to maximize team performance. Great demand for the leader's time and presence requires highly developed stress- and time-management skills.

Style 6: Servant leadership: partner stage: moving from focus on organizational goals and activities towards living in connection with the public through community-building skill development.

Leader Qualities

- Concerned with the quality of interaction in the organization and its impact on society as well as with productivity
- Fosters interdependent governance by peer teams on the basis of agreed-upon values
- Encourages group decision making as a normal process along with mutual responsibility and collegiality

Follower Characteristics

- Willing to take on responsibility
- Lives and works at high levels of trust and relationship
- Well-developed creativity and courage of authenticity

Characteristics of this style:

Starting Point	Well-Developed
Dualistic thinking	Comfortable with paradox
Holds on to power selectively	Powerless
Visible in service	Quiet and unseen in service
Honest	Ethical

Impact of style on group/organization:

Leaders at this level of development have an acute awareness of the rights of all human beings, not just those in the organization. Now decisions are made collaboratively and authority is always used cooperatively. Most essential for sustainability is the capacity to balance involvement in the development of a just and humane organization with ample time for solitude and reflection.

Style 7: Prophetic leader: the universal stage.

Qualities/Characteristics:

This level of leadership is rarely found. Leadership and followership are merged; the concepts becoming meaningless. All activity is interdependent

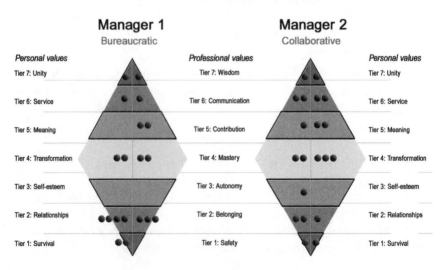

FIGURE 8.7   Leadership profiles.

in nature and global in concern. The focus is on restoring balance between the world of material goods and the needs of each human being; to work on issues related to ecology, human rights, and reconciliation of conflict; along with the creative and humane use of technology. These leaders are rarely seen or heard as their activity is outside formal systems and processes.

Leadership Development Exemplars

Utilizing the I-MAP Model the following values profiles were obtained, see Figure 8.7.

- Manager #1 has an MSN/MBA and 8 years' leadership experience on a surgical critical care unit. Unit is known for high turnover and frequent staffing challenges. Her weighted leadership score placed her in the bureaucratic leadership category.
- Manager #2 has an MSN/MBA and 7 years' leadership experience on a medical critical care unit. Unit is recognized for innovation and low turnover, with a waiting list of nurses wanting to transfer to the unit. Her values cluster placed her in the collaborative manager category.

Upon closer examination, Manager #1 disclosed a childhood with alcoholic parents and the suicide of her husband 2 years earlier. She identified lack of trust in others as a manifestation of her lack of self-trust, and a critical factor in her leadership style. The absence of successful completion of Stage 3 development was a root cause of her management challenges. Her developmental plan included delegating a specific project to a group of staff and working closely with them to assure their success while also building a sense of trust. The following year the survey showed personal values in Stage 3 and a decrease in turnover on her unit. Our personal goals are foundational to professional performance.

BRINGING OUR SOULS TO WORK: PRACTICING FROM A BALANCED CENTER

Growing numbers of professional knowledge workers are expressing a preference for building careers in organizations that have values-based cultures that allow them to make a difference through their work. Such a setting invites people to become all they can be while contributing to the growth and development of colleagues and the institution itself.

Values of all AACN and HHNA Nurses

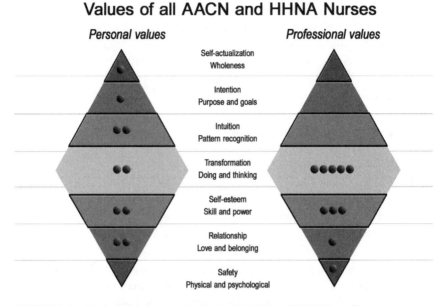

FIGURE 8.8   Professional nursing associations' (AACN and HHNA) profiles.

A values study was conducted with the American Association of Critical Care Nurses and the Home Health Nursing Association utilizing the Seven Levels of Consciousness Model developed by Richard Barrett and Associates (Bodensteiner, 2001). It was designed to explore personal and professional values patterns within and across the two subspecialties. Surveying several hundred nurses nationwide, the results demonstrated that all of the participants had shared values, and a healthy balance in all levels of consciousness in their personal lives. However, not a single one brought values of higher consciousness (levels 5–7, which reflect service, meaning, and making a difference) to the workplace. See Figure 8.8.

The study demonstrated an imbalance in the professional practice environments throughout the country. It suggests that either the organizational structure and bureaucracy of health care organizations does not support higher service goals, or nurses view their job as a means to an end rather than a professional career of service.

While our story is filled with incredible acts of caring and compassion, we also hold the collective memory of systematic oppression and gender discrimination. Nursing has a long and challenging history around its relationships with physicians, health care organizations, and each other (Achterberg, 1990).

Human evolution is replete with a history of widespread trauma and wounding. Our collective consciousness carries the burden of hundreds of millions of people who have experienced the ravages of genocide, human rights violations, racial and ethnic conflicts. Simultaneously, in the past 5 years, new wars, violence, neglect, and weather disasters have added millions of others to the toll of those scarred and wounded (Thompson & O'Dea, 2005).

New ideas and initiatives focused on addressing the intractable conflicts and complex social intergenerational wounds are emerging in every sector of society. There is a global awakening for the need to transition from violence and massive social wounding towards building a framework for a culture committed to peace and wholeness.

Nursing is situated in a strategic position to assist with the social healing of a fractured world in general, and our own discipline in particular. Following the tragedy of 9/11 many parents called in to TV children's show host Mr. Rogers, asking how to help their child. His immediate response was, "keep them focused on the helpers."

Healing of an individual, a discipline, or a world begins with the recognition of the role that mind consciousness plays in the recovery process. Just as medical research has demonstrated the link between mind (thoughts, feelings, and emotions) and body, social healing views the communal group mind as critical to moving forward. We share commonly held images, attitudes, beliefs, and collective traumas, which are instrumental in shaping and creating either the repetitive feedback loop of victim/perpetrator or liberation from it. The work of social healing helps to soften the well-worn identity frames that keep us bound in outworn spaces.

Social nursing-feminine wounds are held in the social body—a shared structure of meaning that bonds the group together. As a result, if true healing is to occur, there must be a transformation of consciousness, a new way of understanding at the personal level the context, content, and possibilities for reconciliation concerning the phenomenon. Simultaneously this must be accompanied by a system-wide transformation of the organizations in which we are nested. The process must be both interactive and interdependent. This calls for an intrinsically holistic approach to social healing, by addressing both its structural and spiritual dimensions.

The health of our discipline, the health of society and the Earth that sustains us all, must take into account all dimensions of our global traumas, from the personal to the political, from the biological to the spiritual. True social healing will require change on many levels. We must explore structures of economics, politics, regulation, and justice, along with social and cultural aspects of the health care field. Simultaneously, we must stay alert to the quality of our individual awareness, our own expressions of compassion in action, the truth of our interdependence, and how we contribute to it (Thurman, 2004).

Social position (race/education/economic status), privilege, and power are concerns of the spirit that must be considered. While we explore central issues with people of power, we must be equally aware of our own attitudes towards and relationship with the many multiskilled workers who carry out support services that assist our daily practice. How do we honor, respect and interact with those who are not us?

Nursing is a universal phenomenon. The global field of nursing can stand together as we extend the responsibility for healing our collective professional wound to the greater whole. However, we must be mindful of the impact that our own privileges may have on others. We must understand the implications of coming from a society with a context for power that includes a legacy of systemic imbalances created through a history of slavery, genocide of native peoples, discriminatory policies, and an ongoing mentality of punitive and retributive actions including war and incarceration. Truth and reconciliation are crucial to understand in every context of our lives.

New understandings occur through a shared dialogue of the heart. Such encounters reveal that space in-between, where a greater knowing and truth reside. Upon the ending of apartheid in South Africa, Desmond Tutu observed that retribution closes any chance for a future. Reconciliation, on the other hand, opens the door for tomorrow. Transitioning from the age-old issues of oppression that have plagued our profession for so long is no easy journey. This complex healing journey requires finding the balance between truth and justice, peace and mercy. It is a multigenerational task rather than an immediate fix. In the end, it is a task for each one of us to accomplish personally. We are then in a position to offer new insights, create a deeper conversation, and give birth to new models and metaphors that will restore wholeness to the profession and the field. Only then will nursing as a collective offer a truly healing presence to the world.

> *When we learn to trust the deep resources of our own being, we discover more than simple renewal. We begin to touch the place where the universe is alive with fresh insight, new possibilities, and supportive resources for realizing our highest ideals. This inner resource flows from an alignment of both heart and mind, making a commitment to the collective human journey through a science of being that flows from an open heart and mind. This generates a positive path for human evolution and genuine progress on planet Earth.*

Unknown teacher

BIBLIOGRAPHY

Achterberg, J. (1990). *Woman as healer: A panoramic survey of the healing activities of women from prehistoric times to present.* Boston: Shambhala.

Barrett, R. (1998). *Liberating the corporate soul: Building a visionary organization.* Woburn, MA: Butterworth-Heinemann.

Benner, P. (1984). *From novice to expert: Excellence and power in clinical nursing practice.* New York: Addison Wesley Publishing Company.

Benner, P., Tanner, C. A., & Chesla, C. A. (1996). *Expertise in nursing practice: Caring, clinical judgment, and ethics.* New York: Springer Publishing, LLC.

Bodensteiner, L. (2001). Decreasing attrition rates across the generations through values alignment. *Seminar for Nurse Managers, 9*(3), 182–187.

Choquette, S. (2000). *True balance: A commonsense guide for renewing your spirit.* New York: Three Rivers.

Coles, R., & Erikson, E. (2000). *The Erik Erikson reader.* New York: W. W. Norton.

Drucker, P. (1999). *Management challenges for the 21st century.* San Francisco: Harper Collins.

Erikson, E. (1980). *Identity and the life cycles.* New York: W. W. Norton.

Hall, B. P. (1986). *The genesis effect: Personal and organizational transformations.* New York: Paulist Press.

Izzo, J. B., & Withers, P. (1996). *Values shift: The new work ethic and what it means for business.* Toronto: Prentice Hall Canada.

Kumar, S. (2004). The dance of choice and choicelessness. *Shift: At the Frontiers of Consciousness, 4* (4), 32–35.

Leddy, S., & Pepper, J. M. (1989). *Conceptual bases of professional nursing* (2nd Ed.). Philadelphia: J. B. Lippincott.

Lehman, B. (2004). The freedom of yes. *Shift: At the Frontiers of Consciousness, 4* (4), 11–13.

Leonard, G. (1992). *Mastery: The keys to success and long-term fulfillment.* New York: Penguin.

Lewis, H. (1991). *A question of values: Six ways we make the personal choices that shape our lives.* San Francisco: HarperCollins.

Maslow, A. H. (1980). *The further reaches of human nature.* New York: Penguin.

Mezirow, J., et al. (1991). *Fostering critical reflection in adulthood: A guide to transformative and emancipatory learning.* San Francisco: Jossey Bass.

Rogers, C. (1980). *A way of being.* New York: Houghton Mifflin.

Thompson, J., & O'Dea, J. (2005). Social healing for a fractured world. *Shift: At the frontiers of consciousness, 7*(3), 10–13.

Thurman, R. (2004). *Infinite life: Seven virtues for living well.* New York: Penguin.

CHAPTER 9

Healing Virtues

Expressions of the Soul

Remember with gratitude the fruits of the labors of others,
Remember the beautiful things seen, heard and felt,
Remember the moments of distress that proved to be groundless,
Remember the new people met who teach true character and human dignity,
Remember the dreams who keep us ever mindful of hopes and goals which
inspire,
Remember the Spirit of the One who seeks us out in our aloneness,
Who gives a sense of assurance that undercuts despair
And confirms life with new courage and abiding hope.

Howard Therman

$\mathbf{A}$s healers, we are living on the edge of a new era where a shift in conscious awareness is moving us beyond thinking and personality, into the deeper world of universal wisdom and the inner wisdom of our soul. Personal character is the individual manifestation of our stage on this soul journey. It is character that creates the context of our life; the spiritual fabric and moral imperative that impels us forward.

Virtuous qualities are character traits of being that emanate from the soulful spark of life that is within each of us. A virtue is a particular dimension of our soul; an order of the angels that is found in all. A manifestation of our conscience, it is a commendable quality or trait, a highly skilled capacity to act. While values are a guiding force for choices and decisions, virtues cannot be created on demand. They are manifestations of our consciousness, the focus from which our behavior emanates when the personality-ego is transcended. An expression of love that radiates from one heart to another, virtues transcend logic and intuition. They flow from the soul as an outpouring of who we are. We uncover and manifest these qualities over time as life experience touches us with joy and wonder, sorrow and pain, *if* we focus on those moments as opportunities for growth.

Little children are completely authentic, with actions guided by instinct and emotions. They listen to the silent promptings of their own integrity from a framework of wholeness. They gather *information* from a multiplicity of sources both formal and exploratory in nature. As they learn to navigate the world and engage in shared relationships through thought, word, and action, their attention gets programmed with *knowledge:* concepts, rules, assumptions, and beliefs. Slowly, simple awareness is replaced with an incessant stream of assumptions and thoughts.

As our attention gets increasingly focused on the information and knowledge in our heads, we no longer perceive the world through the eyes of innocence and unconditional love. We see only that which we have learned to believe, missing the true presence of All-That-Is. The voice of information and knowledge never stops talking, judging, gossiping, and filling our life with background noise and distraction. It sabotages our happiness and keeps us from enjoying the reality of authenticity, truth, and love in the moment. This too, is a stage of development.

The path to *wisdom* is an ongoing movement from the innocence of childhood, through the years of information and knowledge acquisition and management, ever evolving towards increased understanding and higher intelligence. Wisdom is a return to the stage of wonder. However, this time we own a discernment distilled from our lived experience, which turns borrowed knowledge into our own truth. Life once again becomes an expression of our authentic self with a knowing that transcends articulation.

Occasionally we come in contact with something that defies understanding— a moment of *mystery*. When we stand in the presence of the unknowable, we are filled with a sense of awe, wonder, and an illumined knowing that transcends thought. In that moment we are standing on sacred ground, a space pulsating with a disclosure of the truth of All-That-Is.

While our outer purpose is to grow and change over time, our inner purpose is to remember the truth of who we are. Instead of being lost in thinking, we recognize ourselves as the awareness behind the thought. Awareness takes charge from the thinking that has governed our lives, and connects us with our true soul. The creation of meaning is the way in which we use life experiences to transcend limitations.

Teilhard de Chardin suggests we need a "lookout point in the universe" as we launch into the next phase of human evolution. Peaceful existence cannot rely on thinking or reason; we must follow a deeper organic rhythm. In the center of our soul lies our inner wisdom, which will lovingly guide us into each tomorrow as we uncover and manifest the virtues that are ours.

Self-remembering is the soul's journey, the way we use life experiences to grow and deepen as human beings. Moving through the various stages of knowing until we arrive in close communion with our own inner wisdom evolves as we practice the art of remembering. In her compelling book, *Standing Stark*, conscious living teacher Carla Woody gives us ways to live an unencumbered life. She suggests that what we hold inside our minds as true and possible forms the edge of our reality. Building on the pathbreaking work of mythologist Joseph Campbell, she presents the transformational remembering process in five stages (Woody, 2004, pp. 171–178):

1. Sparking is the awakening from an unconscious life, usually slowly and over a period of time. The task is to wake up to the current state of our lives.
2. Separation is a time of unlearning and uncoupling. Examination of jobs, relationships, homes, beliefs—nothing is exempt from this in-depth sorting and releasing.
3. Searching leads to widening choices. Increasingly we explore areas that are new and different, discovering what fits our core *self*.
4. Initiation is the process of assimilation of our increased awareness and new ways of being into our lives. We drop all masks and pretense, appreciate the old life for all its gifts, and step beyond with intent.
5. Re-entry calls us to immersion back into the world in which we live. We are now ready to share, teach, support, and guide others undertaking a similar journey.

Others who have gone before us have left guideposts for our journey from innocence and information to wisdom and wholeness. In their own way each has observed that *expanding personal awareness is the key to wholeness*. Translation of experience into words, metaphors, and stories allows us to share the insight gleaned by others. The following is a collection of observations expressed by patients, professionals, and family caregivers alike. Their role has not been identified, because you will see the universal nature of their articulated wisdom. Focusing questions and growth opportunities are also offered as a guide to prompt reflection on your own healing journey. These insights are shared as a gift of encouragement for your continued journey of remembering.

In a true healing relationship, both heal and both are healed.

Rachel Naomi Remen

PHASE I: INFORMATION—THE WORLD AS MIRROR

It is important to understand that the science and logic we call reality is a manifestation of the world our mind creates, a reflection of our beliefs and our intentions.

Virtue #1: Conscious Living—Living the Examined Life

Focusing questions: Why do you do what you do? What is your intention for helping?

> In truth, no one had ever adequately prepared me for the wonders of [caregiving]: the emotional ups and downs; the spiritual element that can tax one's faith, can shake it to its very foundation; the observation of miracles; and the growth and development that occur beyond one's wildest imagination. In the final analysis, nursing puts us in touch with being human.
>
> M. Patricia Donahue

> I served for many dysfunctional reasons. I served so that you would like me. I became a nurse so that I could look at your problems instead of my own. I served so that I could feel in control. When not in control, I felt an inner anxiety that stemmed from an uncontrollable past. I served so that I could feel needed, since I needed to be needed. I served so that you would give me esteem, because I could not give myself any.
>
> Caryn Summers

> We sometimes speak as if caring did not require knowledge, as if caring for someone, for example, were simply a matter of good intentions or warm regard. But in order to care I must understand the other's needs and I must be able to respond properly to them, and clearly good intentions do not guarantee this. I do not try to help the other grow in order to actualize myself, but by helping the other grow I do actualize myself.
>
> Milton Mayeroff

> I came to [caregiving] without my own thinking; using research or others' ideas as my own, feeling ashamed of thoughts I had about healing, and fearful, believing I didn't have the right to speak up or out. Unaware of my neediness, I was able to use the theories of others and take care of others to shore myself up. I excelled, and my colleagues fed me the definition of myself that I created for them. I never felt full.
>
> David Willard

> What is true healing? And what is the place of the healer within the healing process? In my eighty years, I seemed to experiment with a whole range of answers to these vital questions. Through the process of "discovering the healer," with its leaps of understanding and moments of self-discovery, I have experienced the vital importance of a surrendered heart. When our primary motivation is to be totally available to the life process, any distinction between "healer" and "healee" disappears, and there is only one I AM.
>
> Frances Horn

It is important to gain self/other knowledge as part of spiritual growth and balance—to know yourself and believe in yourself means you can know and believe in God. Knowledge of yourself produces humility, and knowledge of God produces love.

Mother Teresa

Sad that so often [helping] imprisons us, that because of it we find ourselves accomplices to conditions of separateness and division—a world of nurses and patients, social workers and clients, spiritual teachers and seekers, people who know and people who don't. After all, if some of us are busy being helpers there must be others under continuous pressure to be helped. If I stop to think about it, I help out for all kinds of reasons. Maybe it's because I should; it's a matter of responsibility. But there's usually a maze of other motives: a need for self-esteem, approval, status, power; the desire to feel useful, find intimacy, and pay back some debt.

Ram Dass

With modernization, changing social norms create the need to critically examine the paradigms of thought which we were taught by dominant culture to understand our experience. The process of self-reflection has the potential for profoundly changing the way we make sense of the world, other people and ourselves. Transformative learning, in turn, leads to actions that significantly change the character of our interpersonal relationships, the organizations we work in and socialize, and the world itself.

Jack Mezirow

Growth opportunity: Cultivate self-knowledge through the process of reflection. *Reflection in action* requires focused awareness in the moment. One acts reflexively as well as reflectively as the unique needs of the patient are considered along with the scripts of standardization. *Reflection on action* involves a purposeful review of a significant event after it is over, examining of one's own motives and actions along with their impact on the situation and its outcome.

Virtue #2: Vibrant Health—Being the Change You Want to See in the World

Focusing questions: What is your definition of health? How do you manage and model your health beliefs?

Self-care cannot be accomplished without self-love. We need to ask if we feel worthy enough to care for ourselves, even as a priority over caring for others. We are most effective as caregivers when we are centered in our own sense of well-being.

Caryn Summers

For so much of my life I was run by this nagging voice in the back of my head that kept saying, "You're not doing enough! You're not doing enough!"

But now I'm starting to listen to my body a lot more. It needs tender loving care and I'm the only one who can provide that. Even though I always feared that if I took better care of myself it would mean I'd become selfish or self indulgent, I've discovered that's not the case.

Leonard Felder

Some things in life can not be avoided: death, illness, change, personal expectations. What each of them does to us depends a great deal on the way we have allowed ourselves to deal with lesser things. Stability centers us in something greater than ourselves so that nothing lesser than ourselves can possibly sweep us away.

Joan Chittister

When experiencing difficulty in discerning your own needs, it may be helpful to begin by observing what you provide for others. Often we give to other people what we unconsciously know that we need ourselves.

Carmen Renee Berry

Beyond treating the symptom, the physician has the responsibility representing wellness to the patient, of being a totem of wellness rather than a figure associated only with disease.

Dawson Church

To love yourself is to heal yourself.

Course in Miracles

Health is not equivalent to happiness, surfeit, or success. It is foremost a matter of being wholly one with whatever circumstances we find ourselves in. Even our death is a healthy event if we fully embrace the fact of our dying. . . . The issue is awareness, of living in the present. Whatever our present existence consists of, if we are at one with it, we are healthy.

Elizabeth Kubler-Ross

If I don't do me, I don't get done.

Jacquelyn Small

Every day is another chance to discover more about yourself—what are your strengths and limitations as a caregiver; what are you really like as a family member or friend; what are you learning about your own ability to express love, patience, and caring; and what are you discovering about your priorities in life?

Leonard Felder

Growth opportunity: Cultivate healthy balance in your life. Identifying and managing your personal issues are as critical to vibrant health as diet and nutrition—it is an ongoing process of discovery, forgiveness, and release. Pay attention to little tugs and resistances and discern when you felt like that before. What is it stirring up for you? How can you bless it, transcend it, and move on?

Virtue #3: Focused Clarity—Seeing the Whole Rather Than the Hole

Focusing questions: What is your personal accountability in any situation, in your life, to all of life?

Our most profound growth comes during our most painful times. Becoming aware of the difficulty is the first step in finding the solution. Once we acknowledge our despair and admit that we are powerless, we become empowered. Once we admit that our lives are unmanageable, we no longer have to pretend to be in control. By stating our confusion, we make the first move toward clarity. When denial stops, the process of healing begins. In the center of chaos lies the promise of clarity.

Caryn Summers

The best gift a serious illness gives us is the ability to become "clear" . . . to accept our troubled areas—fear, doubt, and love ourselves in spite of them. The best gift you can give yourself and others is the gift of clarity. It takes fear, doubt, etc. and makes them disappear. Go inside to uncover the hidden mysteries of your self and then jump on the outside to see how your "healing" can begin the "healing" for someone else. GET CLEAR! I would rather be clear for 1 day than to live to be 100 in the dark. The gift I would give myself would outlive me because it would change the consciousness of those I love most. That is one of the most significant purposes of living and we often don't even see it. Illness can be the ultimate gift if you surrender, embrace and love all that it brings into your life for better or worse . . . because you see there never has been or will be a worse. When you get clear on this all else will be just as it should.

Kristi Welch

It's more about living life well than keeping the law perfectly. . . . It involves a conscious gathering of the wisdom of others who can encourage us and help us scrutinize our own choices for their value and their valor. Learn to see what you are looking at and then say what you see. Looking is so difficult in our culture which is highly technological and intent on fixing on what is not broken.

Joan Chittister

What is to give light must endure burning.

Vicktor Frankl

I have a clear choice between life and death, between reality and fantasy, between health and sickness. I have to become responsible—responsible for mistakes as well as accomplishments.

Eileen Mayhew

We labor under the myth that it is the ministrations of health-care providers that cure or heal people. This is simply an illusion, a product of faulty logic. The assumption is that if a patient gets well after surgery, she gets well because of surgery. The reality is that surgery does not cure/heal. Drugs do not cure/heal. Acupuncture, or crystals, or homeopathy do not cure/ heal. The person who undergoes the surgery, or takes the drug, or receives the alternative treatment must heal herself. Any or all of the above-named ministrations may be necessary to remove barriers to self-healing or to stimulate it, but they are not sufficient causes for healing.

Janet F. Quinn

Have the courage to act instead of react.

Darlene Larson Jenks

Being stuck in the past is just another form illusion can take. The message seems to be: Complete, with honesty, whatever is bothering you, and then . . . stop looking back.

Jacquelyn Small

Life is tragic, but not necessarily serious. We are small people, here for a while. The sounds will soon cover over our seemingly important enterprises. Let's do our best, respect each other, and hope that someone's passage is the better for our existence.

John Neil

Growth opportunity: A choice-point exists where past and future overlap. Cultivate your decision-making capacity without wearing dark or rose-colored glasses. Release fears created in past experiences and expectations for future outcomes. Let the moment guide your course of action by seeing it for what it is and trusting the process of life towards greater good.

PHASE II: KNOWLEDGE—LIVED EXPERIENCE AS TEACHER

I may have misinformation, but I never have a misexperience.

De Lorian

Virtue #4: Reverence for All Life—Holding an Interconnected View of the Universe

Focusing questions: What comprises your worldview? How are things related and how do they work?

Each thing on earth holds a spark of life. Seeing and appreciating its beauty is the recognition of our shared spark from the creator. All things are our relatives.

Wanigi Waci

For me there is a reverence for life. It means enjoying the sunshine, the rain, a dust storm, walking down the city street, and looking to see the pleasure, to smell the fresh air. It means bringing the country with me to the city. It's working hard in my garden. It's reading a good book. It's being with people I enjoy. It's even being with people I don't enjoy. It's learning to choose. It's learning I can't care for everyone. It's having an obligation not to cause pain in this life and to ease it when I can.

Nola Pennert

Alone I am what I am, but in community I have the chance to become everything that I can be. Humility is a basic awareness of my relationship to the world and my connectedness to all its circumstances. . . . There is no haughtiness, distance, sarcasm, put downs, airs of importance or disdain. The ability to deal with our own and others limitations flows from the recognition that God is in life, relieving us from being in charge of the universe. This brings serenity and hope, inner peace and energy.

Joan Chittister

There is in every true heart a spark of heavenly fire,
Which lies dormant in the broad daylight of prosperity;
But which kindles up and beams and blazes
In the dark hour of adversity.

Anonymous Proverb

We are healed of a suffering only by experiencing it to the full.

Marcel Proust

To understand ourselves and our place in the world, we might pay more attention to the natural laws, to the life cycle of animals and plants. Nature reflects the Universal Laws. Oversee its working in the habits of birds, the cycles of plants, and the instincts of reptiles and mammals. All teach the secrets of life. Watch the coming and going of clouds, the waxing and waning of the moon, the rising and setting of the sun. They reveal the natural order of creation. Everything is right when there is neither too much nor too little for the time and place.

Harold Klemp

Loving others is an expression of our love for God.

Mother Teresa

I ask, how would nature solve this? I try to think like nature to find the right questions. You don't invent answers; you reveal the answers from nature. In nature the answers to all our problems already exist.

Dr. Jonas Salk

When we learn both to take and to give, we can move into a flow of giving and receiving that is love's essence—reciprocity. In this way, the flow of energy does not go just one way, but both. I give to you and you to me and we both fully receive the energy. Christ said to "love your neighbor as yourself." Sacrifice, however, has been misinterpreted as loving your neighbor instead of yourself.

Carol S. Pearson

The fragrance of the rose lingers on the hand of the giver.

Unknown teacher

Growth opportunity: Cultivate an appreciation for beauty in music, the arts, and nature. Explore the new discoveries in space, quantum science, and technology as well as economics, social sciences, and spirituality. Become informed about environmental issues and practice a simplistic lifestyle of "living lightly on the earth."

Virtue #5: Authentic Presence—Being Real So Others Can Show Up Also

Focusing questions: What is your life story? How does it enrich and limit your continuing unfolding?

When one is a stranger to oneself, then one is estranged from others . . . if one is out of touch with oneself, then one cannot touch others.

Anne Morrow Lindbergh

Authentic service can be seen in the nurse who has nurtured herself, the healer who has been healed. It is the service we hear when the nurse can speak from her heart to the patient these simple and humble words, "I am here." Let's heal together."

Caryn Summers

Life is lived in cycles of seven years. Every seven years all cells are replaced in your body, and they are genetically influenced by your ancestors. What happens in your life emotionally and spiritually also touches seven generations. As the middle [fourth] generation, your influence extends from you back to your parents, your grandparents and great-grandparents. It also goes out from you to your children, grandchildren and great-grandchildren. Healing efforts made on your part will also heal them, while injuries you create will also hurt them. Remember the accountability you have to seven generations each time you make a decision.

Wanigi Waci

First try to discover your own childhood, then take the experience seriously. . . . Try to feel, and help the patient to feel . . . study the history of childhood. . . . Therapy has to open you as well as the patient for feeling in your life. It has to awaken you from a sleep.

Alice Miller

The most elusive knowledge of all is self-knowledge.

Mirra Komarovsky

When you look upon another and feel great love towards them, or when you contemplate beauty in nature and something within you responds deeply, close your eyes for a moment and feel the essence of that love or beauty, inseparable from who you are, your true nature. The outer form is a temporary reflection of what you are within, in your essence. That is why love and beauty can never leave you, although all outer forms will.

Eckhart Tolle

To me, healing is releasing from the past. It is retraining my mind so as not to see the shadow of the past on anyone. It is learning not to make interpretations of people's behavior or motives. It is letting go of the desire to want to change another person. It is letting go of expectations, assumptions, and the desire to control or manipulate another person.

Gerald Tampolsky

The curriculum of service provides us with information about our strengths and our weaknesses; we discover how these contribute to genuinely helpful service. Each time we drop our masks and meet heart-to-heart, reassuring one another simply by the quality of our presence, we experience a profound bond which we intuitively understand is nourishing everyone.

Ram Dass

What we grew up with we learned;
What we learned, we practiced;
And what we practiced, we became.

Ernie Larsen

Growth opportunity: Become familiar with your life story. Know your own attitudes, values, and beliefs so that you do not project them onto others. Visit friends and relatives to get other perspectives. Know your family of origin and recognize the patterns you inherited. Purposefully choose which ones to maintain and which to forgive and transcend. Be the example you want your children to become.

Virtue #6: Creative Imagination—Opening Space for Spontaneous Creation to Emerge

Focusing questions: What rules govern your reality? How do you transcend them?

Healing in the future must involve major shifts in the way we think about health and illness. The focus of a health-care system must be on facilitating wholeness, which means facilitating right relationship. The techniques are beside the point. What must occur is twofold: the revaluing of the feminine principle and its ways, and the empowerment of individuals and communities to create their own health and healing.

Janet Quinn

Life is either a daring adventure or nothing.

Helen Keller

It is time to break free of our overly serious approach to life and laugh, have fun, cultivate frivolity and joy. We [helpers] need to learn how to say "Yes!"—to having fun, to going on adventures, to attending spiritual retreats, to spontaneous outings, to developing our artistic talents, to listening to music, to reading enjoyable books, to soaking in bubble baths, to exercising regularly, to filling our homes with cut flowers and beauty and art.

Carmen Renee Berry

Every atom is striving continually to manifest more life; all are intelligent, and all are seeking to carry out the purpose for which they were created. Life is a mystery until we begin to understand that we can be the creators of our own world and that, in truth, what we are today is a creation of that which we have made from the past.

Paul Twitchell

Artistic creation, sports, dance, teaching, counseling—mastery in any field of endeavor implies that the thinking mind is either no longer involved at all or at least is taking second place. A power and intelligence greater than you and yet one with you in essence takes over. There is no decision-making process anymore; spontaneous right action happens. . . . Mastery of life is the opposite of control. You become aligned with the greater consciousness. It acts, speaks, does the work.

Eckhart Tolle

Only those who dare truly live.

Ruth P. Freedman

Develop a sense of humor, and as challenges come up, you begin to draw on your creativity. You find solutions that would never have occurred to you before. Life becomes more fun—you have a more adventuresome life. You get put into situations you would not have been in before, because you are going one step beyond yourself. And as you get yourself in trouble, you also have help to get out of it, because as you learn to work with your own resources, you are developing self-mastery.

Harold Klemp

Take two jokes and call me in the morning.

Unknown teacher

Thought creates form, but it is feeling that gives vitality to the thought.

Unknown teacher

Growth opportunity: Transcend the silent rules and assumptions that govern your reality by observing nature and young children at play. Reclaim your birthright: a deep sense of awe, wonder, and discovery fostered by non–ego-dominated exploration. Refine the ability to identify thought patterns blocked and stunted by desire or intellect. Open space for spontaneous creation to emerge by increasing your ability to see potential and possibility in every situation rather than stopping at a scripted standard.

PHASE III: WISDOM—PRESENT MOMENT AS GUIDE

Wisdom is not a product of thought. The deep knowing that is wisdom arises through the simple act of giving someone your full attention. Attention is primordial intelligence.

Eckhart Tolle

Virtue #7: Courageous Vigilance—Bearing Witness to Suffering With Merciful Detachment

Focusing questions: What is hard for you to look at or acknowledge? How do you determine and establish boundaries in an encounter?

Detachment doesn't mean not to get involved; it means to not let outer circumstances throw off your inner balance. We will all have a certain amount of pain and pleasure, but will not let it overly affect our emotional balance if we are detached from fear. Only when fear is in control of those two poles is your life attached to its physical, mental and spiritual possessions. Give up fear and you need never give up another thing in your life. Great joys can become yours, balanced by what sorrows need to be in your life.

Harold Klemp

Those who do not know how to weep with their whole heart don't know how to laugh either.

Golda Meir

Unless we as healers are willing to confront our own pain and darkness, we can never be truly open to that joining of energy with our patients that is necessary for the fullest healing process to take place for both.

Niravni Payne

The abuse of power is solving problems for people that belong to them.

Stewart Block

No excuse is good enough for neglecting to reach out and embrace our loved ones while they are still alive. Death can come when we least expect it, so we must take every opportunity to give our love [and presence] to those around us. The time is now!

Barry and Joyce Vissell

To detach means to give others the freedom to grow through their own mistakes and experiences. It is not feeling responsible for others, but rather allowing others to learn self-responsibility.

Caryn Summers

You heal a brother by recognizing his worth.

Course in Miracles

To study the Way is to study the Self.
To study the Self is to forget the Self.
To forget the Self is to be enlightened by all things.
To be enlightened by all things is to remove the barrier
Between Self and Other.

Dogen Zenji

Trust in the other to grow and in my own ability to care gives me courage to go into the unknown, but it is also true that without the courage to go into the unknown such trust would be impossible.

Milton Mayeroff

Courage is the price that life extracts for peace. Courage is the last uncrowded place in the Universe.

Amelia Earhart

Growth opportunity: Cultivate your dark side. Until there is self-awareness, unconscious projection and role-playing makes up a large part of human interaction. By letting go of your resistance to the hard things in life you become vulnerable. This softens the hard and rigid parts of your soul, making you available to yourself and others. By being at risk you will discover and share your true essential nature, which is the same essence in all of humanity.

Virtue #8: Elegant Timing—Practicing Effortless Learning and Living

Focusing questions: What prompts you to act? How much effort is expended for the outcome obtained?

There have been great leaders such as Lincoln and King across history. While there have been many able men, at certain times the personality, the needs and values of society align in such a way that the individual is literally propelled into a leadership position. Timing is the essence of wisdom. If it is too difficult, and you find yourself pulling or pushing, the time is not right. Patience and discernment are the antidotes to poor timing.

Emil Erikson

Each person faces a time of danger and a time of potential transformation. It's not for any of us to judge their response. It is for us to "be there" for them, not necessarily to "do" for them.

Rraeme Amontee

You must be careful to do what is appropriate and evolutionary for the other. Otherwise you become a compulsive cornucopia, burying someone under all the gifts you are pouring out. Your apparent generosity is not always appreciated, and indeed may be deeply resented.

Jean Houston

An easy litmus test can determine whether one is giving or enabling. If, when we give, we feel either used or smugly superior; it is time to look at what really is going on. Healthy giving is respectful of both the giver and the receiver.

Carol S. Pearson

There is a divine plan of good at work in my life. I will let go and let it unfold.

Ruth P. Freedman

Effortless learning and effortless living occurs when you quit striving. As a Harvard student I applied myself but got mediocre grades. One huge college assignment was given in comparative literature. I put it off because of its difficulty until the night before it was due. Rather than reading the thick volumes of Freud and Durkheim, I literally skimmed through the books, underlining anything that leaped out as interesting. I began to notice that here and there some of their ideas were opposed or in alignment. I marked those places and typed whatever came to me about the two. I had no choice; I had to do it. It was interesting and fun to write. I was relaxed, enjoying it because I knew I was going to get an F. That paper was the first and only A+ that I ever got at Harvard.

Gary Zukav

Care-giving and rescuing are a lot different. Rescuing can make the rescuer feel good; but it might not make the patient feel good.

Dave Morris

I slept and dreamt that life was joy,
I awoke and saw that life was service,
I acted and behold, service was joy.

Rabindranath Tagore

There is a thin line between giving and unhealthy "enabling" (i.e., supporting someone else's dependency or irresponsibility). Sometimes we persist in giving to people who use our gifts and energy only to help themselves continue in a destructive pattern.

Carlos Petres

Growth opportunity: Cultivate the capacity to identify the subtle in all things. Intuition is the recognition of pattern by sensing slight shifts leading towards disruption. Develop trust in your own wisdom in the moment and respond in real time instead of waiting for affirmation from external experts. Be present in the now, for it holds all the information needed for right timing.

Virtue #9: Compassionate Caring—Experiencing Nonjudgment and Forgiveness for All

Focusing questions: How do you demonstrate caring to others, to yourself? What problems are yours to solve?

Nothing may be more important than being gentle with ourselves. Whether we're professionals working a sixty-hour week or simply family members called upon to care daily for a sick relative, facing suffering continuously is no small task. We learn the value of recognizing our limits, forgiving ourselves our bouts of impatience or guilt, acknowledging our own needs. We see that to have compassion for others we must have compassion for ourselves.

Ram Dass

Caring for others is a deepening process. We begin with sympathy; "I feel sorry for you." It is an act of separation for you are experiencing something I am not. Then comes the state of empathy; "I am one with you, I can relate." In this space we find our similarity and shared connection. This is followed by a mature state of compassion; "I am distressed for you, myself and all who are in a similar state, including the earth." Here we are at-one with the world, and the depth of our emotion compels us to social action— to correct the injustice against all beings.

Matthew Fox

It is not how much you do but how much love you put into the doing and sharing with others that is important. Try not to judge people. If you judge others then you are not giving love.

Mother Teresa

As our understanding of our own suffering deepens, we become available at deeper levels to those we would care for. We are less likely to project suffering that does not exist or deny that which does. We're much more sensitive and alert to the nuances of human pain. Compassion and pity are very different. Whereas compassion reflects the yearning of the heart to merge and take on some of the suffering, pity is a controlled set of thoughts designed to assure separateness. Compassion is the spontaneous response of life, pity, the involuntary reflex of fear.

Ram Dass

When we see another person with problems, we can have compassion; but we understand that somewhere down the path these problems have emerged by his own efforts. While we can offer compassion and support, we must let him have the freedom to experience his troubles. People of good intentions—who are often short on patience—sometimes forget the Law of Non-interference.

Harold Klemp

All the healing techniques in the world won't really help unless love goes with them.

Louise L. Hay

Caring is the antithesis of simply using the other person to satisfy one's own needs.

Milton Mayeroff

No one ever becomes a perfect being. There is always one more step towards wholeness. We always seek, but never find, completion.

Harold Klemp

Growth opportunity: Cultivate the capacity for nonjudgment and forgiveness of yourself and others. As you surrender the striving for perfection, you quit putting impossible demands on every situation, person, place, or event. Your life, and the experience of others whom you touch, becomes more harmonious and peaceful. A state of nonresistance opens you to universal awareness, which is vastly greater than your human mind. You move naturally with the flow and timing of events, enriched by respect for the resilience of the human spirit—and the divine.

PHASE IV: MYSTERY—THE UNKNOWN AS INSPIRATION

Become at ease with the state of "not knowing." This takes you beyond the mind which is always trying to conclude and interpret . . . Truth is far more all-encompassing than mind could ever comprehend.

Eckhart Tolle

Virtue #10: Learned Ignorance—Releasing the Need for Certainty and Predictability

Focusing questions: How do you discern the lesson offered in each situation? What memory or belief may be released or reframed?

An attitude of not having anything further to learn is incompatible with caring.

Milton Mayeroff

The reward, the real grace of conscious service . . . is the opportunity not only to help relieve suffering but to grow in wisdom, experience greater unity, and have a good time while we're doing it.

Ram Dass

I don't think we can stand back and look at ourselves and our culture and the way we live in the world, raping the world, without feeling sad. I try to see life like a lake. The anger and the politics and the bitching and the back-biting and essence of humanizing comes from the deep, dark blue waters underneath. That's where the dolphins and the whales swim. That's where the mysteries are.

Grace Greer

The body knows and the soul knows: only our minds can lie.

Jacquelyn Small

Being a good teacher requires a willingness to take the risk of inviting open dialogue, knowing I can never predict where it is going to take us. I can then see my student's life more clearly than they do, opening a capacity to look beyond their initial self-presentation, helping them see themselves more clearly.

Parker Palmer

The longer I practice medicine, the less sure I am of the dividing line between healer and those in need of healing. Patients whose overwhelming physical problems made me feel useless have taught me volumes about the true nature of my calling, thereby restoring my faith in myself as a doctor.

Bernie Siegel

The harder a person struggles to achieve some goal, the more difficulty he will have to overcome; difficulty caused at least in part, by the strain of his effort. When your attention leaves your mind and moves into the Now, there is an alertness. . . . Such clarity, such simplicity. No room for problem-making. Just this moment as it is.

Eckhard Tolle

One cannot have wisdom without living life.

Dorothy McCall

I have learned to stand back and let the divine work through me. It is facilitated by adopting a certain attitude of curious, childlike devotion. Many people seek this state but the urgency of their physical needs causes tension and fear, closing the channel between themselves and the Spirit.

Competition intensifies the attitude of tension; tension springs from fear; fear rises out of excessive self-love; excessive self-love cuts one off from the qualities leading to satisfaction, happiness, new insights and growth.

Lai Tsi

We each choose our own state of conscious knowing. We make our own worlds. Life carries all people and beings onward to the expansion of consciousness. Across our lifespan, through the use of experience and reflection on that experience, we move from innocence to disillusionment, and then on to conscious innocence.

Phyllis Jones

Growth opportunity: Cultivate the capacity for humility. Recognize that we do not always know or have the answers. Release the need for certainty and predictability, reveling in the true wonder of the moment. Develop an ability to trust and move forward even, especially, when we do not know the how or why of a situation or opportunity. Recognizing and acknowledging what we do not know is the beginning of freedom.

Virtue #11: Active Surrender—Utilizing the Power of Paradox

Focusing questions: What opposing energies are present in this situation? Where is the middle ground?

We must want to be human as well as efficient; to be loving as well as informed; to be caring as well as knowledgeable; to be happy as well as respected. Attendant listening and watching teaches us critical discernment; it evaluates everything, not in the light of what is good for me, but in the light of what is best for all of us. It brings us to growth, to truth and the holy responsibility for the lives of the entire human community.

Joan Chittister

You must learn to be still in the midst of activity and to be vibrantly alive in repose.

Indira Gandhi

Here in the intensive neonatal care unit you see the incredible beauty and the unbearable pain. And you have to figure out how to be with both.

A nurse

It was in the darkness that I found the light. It was in the pain that I found the gain. It was in the dying that I found the life. It was in the aloneness that I found the need of prayer. And it is through the love of God that I found meaning in my life.

A patient

Never try to force results. The more you try to put your imaginative powers upon something in concentrated effort, the less you can do it. Outcome is concerned with imagining and feeling. What you imagine you must feel— therefore the negative impact of striving is more likely to be effective than vivid imagining because the negative has strong feeling with it.

Harold Klemp

The woundedness in each of us connects us in trust. My woundedness evokes your healer, and your woundedness evokes my healer. Then the two healers can collaborate together.

Rachel Naomi Remen

The reason you cannot earn your worth is because you are already worthy. All you can do is accept what is already yours.

Carmen Renee Berry

The beauty of the world has two edges, one of laughter, one of anguish, cutting the heart asunder.

Virginia Woolf

Wounding is the traditional training ground for the healer. Those who have, through accident or illness, vividly confronted the reality of their own death often return to life with a renewed sense of wonder and strength.

Jean Houston

True selflessness is not the abandonment of self, but rather the surrender of selfish motives. The result of this surrender is self love, or self-esteem. We experience our preciousness and value and reach out from that centered place of love, serving authentically.

Caryn Summers

Growth opportunity: Bring balance to complex situations by utilizing the power of paradox. Cultivate the ability to simply be with an event, releasing the need for control. With your intuitive presence identify the polarities and seek the point of connection where the passive middle lies. Here is the point of reconciliation, the space from which new order will emerge and form.

Virtue #12: Mindful Awareness—Stepping Out of the Mind's Contents Into the Moment With Fresh Eyes

Focusing questions: What do you hear when you listen with your inner ear? What do you see when you look through eyes of discernment?

The equivalent of external noise is the inner noise of thinking. The equivalent of external silence is inner stillness. But what is wisdom, and where is it to be found? Wisdom comes with the ability to be still. Just look and just listen. No more is needed. Being still, looking, and listening activates the non-conceptual intelligence within you. Let stillness direct your words and actions.

Eckhart Tolle

The heart does speak most eloquently if we listen with our inner ear. Nursing reaches out to the hearts of others to assist as midwives in the birthing of new consciousness. Nurses have frequent opportunities to facilitate the transformation of the experience of discomfort and disease into one of growth, renewal and opportunity. Let the heart speak clearly, and it will touch the world around!

Susanne Davis

When we learn to be where we are, we gain perspective on life. Yesterday loses its hold on us and tomorrow loses its allure. . . . Mindfulness makes the present, present, and gives us back the energy that endless worry and constant calculation drain. It concentrates what has become scattered and brings us home to ourselves.

Joan Chittister

If we are willing to examine the agitation of our own minds and look just beyond it, we quite readily find entry into rooms that hold surprising possibilities: a greater inner calm, sharper concentration, deeper intuitive understanding, and an enhanced ability to hear one another's heart. Such an inquiry turns out to be critical in the work of helping others.

Ram Dass

Learn to get in touch with silence within yourself and know that everything in this life has a purpose. There are no mistakes, no coincidences. All events are blessings given to us to learn from.

Elizabeth Kubler-Ross

People who cannot live comfortably with silence can never live comfortably with noise. Silence and inactivity is a frightening thing: it leaves us at the mercy of the noise within. Silence invites us to depth . . . it heals what hoarding and running will not touch.

Joan Chittister

The longest journey is the journey inward, for he who has chosen his destiny has started upon his quest for the source of his being.

Dag Hammarsjkold

When you meet anyone, remember it is a holy encounter. Thoughtfulness, the kindly regard for others, is the beginning of holiness.

Mother Teresa

When the higher incorporates the lower into its service, the nature of the lower is transformed into that of the higher.

Meister Eckhart

To heal is to live one's life as a prayer, accepting our natural state of pure joy and happiness, peace and love, and extending that to all life.

Gerald Tampolsky

Growth opportunity: Cultivate planned moments for inner silence and meditation. Create moments of silent solitude so your inner wisdom can be heard. Learn to be still in the midst of chaos by being alert for spiritually meaningful moments in your active life. Live in the now by being totally present, body, mind, and spirit. Now is the only thing that is real.

Never forget that you are not in the world; the world is in you. Remember who you are. When anything happens to you, take the experience inward. Creation will bring you constant hints and clues about your role as a co-creator. Be aware of them; absorb them. Your soul is metabolizing experience as surely as your body is metabolizing food.

Deepak Chopra

BIBLIOGRAPHY

Berry, C. (1988). *When helping you is hurting me: Escaping the messiah trap.* New York: Harper and Row.

Campbell, P. (1985). *Bio-spirituality: Focusing as a way to grow.* Chicago: Loyola University Press.

Donahue, P. (1989). *Nursing: The finest art.* Boston: Mosby.

Dossey, L. (1982). *Space, time and medicine.* Boston: Shambhala.

Houston, J. (1987). *The search for the beloved.* Houston, TX: Jeremy P. Tarcher.

Klemp, H. (2002). *The spiritual laws of life.* Minneapolis, MN: Eckcankar.

Koerner, J. (2003). *Mother heal myself: An intergenerational healing journey between two worlds.* Santa Rosa, CA: Crestport.

Kubler-Ross, E. (1986). *Death: The final stages of growth.* Englewood Cliffs, NJ: Prentice-Hall.

Liberman, J. (1987). *Light: The medicine of the future.* New York: Parabola.

Mayeroff, M. (1991). *On caring.* New York: Harper and Row.

Mother Teresa. (1996). *Meditations from a simple path.* New York: Ballantine.

Newman, M. (1986). *Health as expanding consciousness.* New York. National League for Nursing.

Palmer, P. (1998). *The courage to teach: Exploring the inner landscape of a teacher's life.* San Francisco: Jossey-Bass.

Pearson, C. S. (1986). *The hero within: Six archetypes we live by.* New York: Harper and Row.

Peck, S. (1978). *The road less traveled.* Denver, CO: Simon and Schuster.

Prophet, M. L., & Prophet, E. C. (2001). *The masters and the spiritual path.* Corwin Springs, MT: Summit University Press.

Small, J. (1982). *Transformers: The therapists of the future.* Marina del Bay, CA: DeVorss.

Summers, C. (1993). *Inspirations for caregivers.* Mount Shasta, CA: Commune-A-Key.

Tolle, E. (1999). *Practicing the power of now.* Novato, CA: New World Library.

Tolle, E. (2003). *Stillness speaks.* Novato, CA: New World Library.

Tolle, E. (2005). *A new Earth: Awakening to your life's purpose.* New York: Penguin.

Woody, C. (2004). *Standing stark: The willingness to engage.* Prescott, AZ: Kenosis.

CHAPTER 10

Healing Web
Weaving the Web of Life

We need to stop asking about the meaning of life, and instead to think of ourselves as those who are being questioned by life—daily and hourly. One answer must consist, not in talk and meditation, but in right action and in right conduct. Life ultimately means taking the responsibility to find the right answer to its problems and to fulfill the task which it constantly sets for each individual. These tasks, and therefore the meaning of life, differs from person to person and from moment to moment.

Vicktor Frankl

The offerings of this book have provided a number of concepts and theories regarding the nature of life and its ultimate meaning. This final chapter is an effort to provide a model that allows you to weave these differing ideas and activities into a meaningful tapestry for your own life. Guidance for this effort is taken from the wisdom and lore of the First Nations.

A Message from the Hopi Elders:
You have been telling the people that this is the Eleventh Hour
Now you must go back and tell the people that this is The Hour
Here are the things that must be considered:
Where are you living?
What are you doing?
What are your relationships?
Are you in right relation?
Where is your water?
Know your garden
It is time to speak your Truth
Create your community

Be good to each other
And do not look outside yourself for the leader
This could be a good time!
There is a river flowing now very fast
It is so great and swift that there are those who will be afraid
They will try to hold on to the shore
They will feel like they are being torn apart, and they will suffer greatly
Know the river has its destination
The elders say we must let go of the shore, push off toward the middle of the river.
Keep our eyes open, and our heads above the water.
See who is there with you and celebrate.
At this time in history, we are to take nothing personally, least of all ourselves!
For the moment we do, our spiritual growth and journey comes to a halt.
The time of the lonely wolf is over
Gather yourselves!
Banish the word struggle from your attitude and vocabulary.
All that we do now must be done in a sacred manner and in celebration.
We are the ones we have been waiting for.

The Elders of the Hopi Nation
Oraibi, Arizona

First Nations lore tells the story of Spiderwoman. A great flood fell upon the earth, and she wove a large web. Casting it across the waters, many climbed on and floated to safety. She is the creator of the web of life, which hovers on the edge of chaos.

Evolutionary biologist Stuart Kauffman and his colleagues at the Santa Fe Institute in New Mexico studied complex living systems and the role chaos plays within them (Kauffman, 1993). He discovered that a wide variety of living systems, from neural networks to ecosystems, functioned as cyclical binary networks. At the edge of chaos these binary networks develop a "frozen core" of elements that create "walls of consistency" that grow across the entire system, partitioning the network into separate islands of changing elements. The space between the walls is filled with chaos. Living systems reside on the border at the edge of chaos, rather than in the stable and frozen core. Natural selection favors and sustains living systems "at the edge of chaos" because they are best able to coordinate complex and flexible behavior, best able to adapt and evolve.

WEAVING THE WEB OF YOUR LIFE

Quantum physics shows that outside of relationship there is nothing, that we become only in relationship. People who have significant relationships and connections in their lives enjoy greater health than those who live in isolation. Research shows that social support, comprised of a core of 50 to 100 significant relationships, creates the foundation for a meaningful life. Further, it found that 26% of all Americans list loneliness as a central theme in their lives (Pilisuk & Parks, 1989). Weaving a web of connections and maintaining their health and vibrancy is the key to a meaningful life.

Like Spiderwoman, we each weave our own web of life (Bunkers et al., 1992; Larson et al., 1993). As we follow her example we are able to consciously choose processes and relationships that allow for an expansive and exhilarating existence, or we can get stuck in an immovable space that does not attract the things that give us life (Capra, 1996). The process of web-weaving involves five distinct phases:

I. Foundational lines—self-organizing: All natural systems create their own world through a process of self-organization. The pattern of organization gives a unique shape and identity to the entity. Spiderwoman selects a place to weave her web that is sheltered enough from the natural elements to maintain its integrity while being exposed enough to attract and take in the things essential to sustain her life. The edges we select for our living space are the elements necessary to organize and create the *context* for a whole and balanced life. See Figure 10.1.

Five major elements must be present to build and maintain a foundation of health. Please consider the following in your own life:

1. Personal life: home/environment/education/resources
2. Vibrant health: physical/mental/emotional/spiritual
3. Social relationships: family/friends/coworkers/community
4. Meaningful career: skills/continuous learning/ teamwork/mastery
5. Authentic presence: personal power/empowerment/leadership/service

II. Support line—self-referencing: Living systems pass through stages and cycles, each one referencing off its central core to replicate itself in higher order of complexity, becoming more of its true essence. Spiderwoman weaves a strong central plumb line, which holds and sustains the structure and weight of the web and all its activities for the duration of its existence. She moves back and forth from the plumb line to the edges, casting the fine filaments of her web while always reinforcing this central core.

The central core for humankind, the *values and beliefs* that reflect our level of consciousness, influence the choices that guide the actions of our lives. As

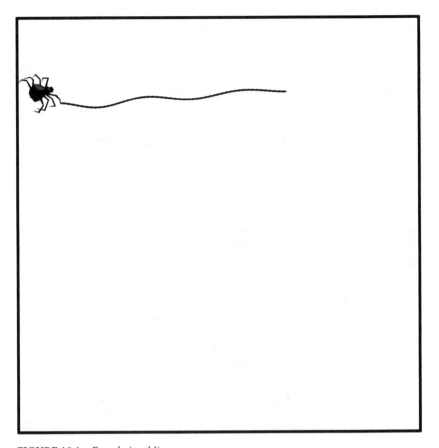

FIGURE 10.1   Foundational lines.

we engage and reflect on our experiences, our values deepen and the core strengthens. See Figure 10.2.

A balanced set of values includes seven stages of consciousness woven into a strong central core. Become familiar with your current values, and those you aspire to develop:

1. Surviving—security
2. Connecting—relationships
3. Feeling—emotions
4. Doing—mastery—*transforming*
5. Knowing—wisdom
6. Being—service
7. Unifying—wholeness

III. Radial lines—self-regulating: Feedback loops are essential for self-balancing: self-reinforcing (positive) and self-balancing (negative) exchanges in

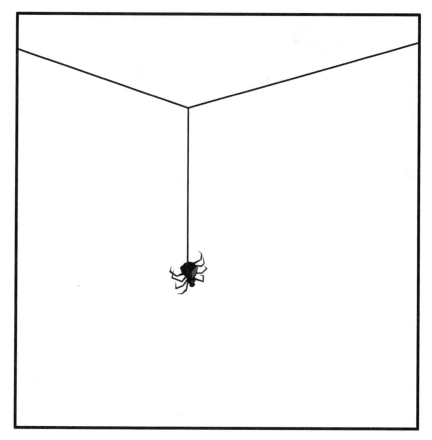

FIGURE 10.2   Support line.

our relationships and experiences help us adjust and adapt in dynamic fashion to all elements of our life. Spiderwoman casts specific threads to various areas of the environment to secure her web, some on immovable objects like concrete or tree trunks, others more flexible, such as a small twig on the periphery of a bush. The pattern and length of these relational lines create the expanse and flexibility of the framework for her weaving. Some are short and close, while others are longer with larger space in between. With combined strength and flexibility, she adjusts and adapts her relationships to her environment and things ensnared in her web, based on what is required to maximize efficiency.

Humankind also creates and explores *relationships* of varying purpose and length, which form and inform the personality, guiding the depth of exchange between the outer world of our experiences and the inner world of our spirits. Both positive and negative encounters give feedback with which to learn, evaluate, adapt, and progress. See Figure 10.3.

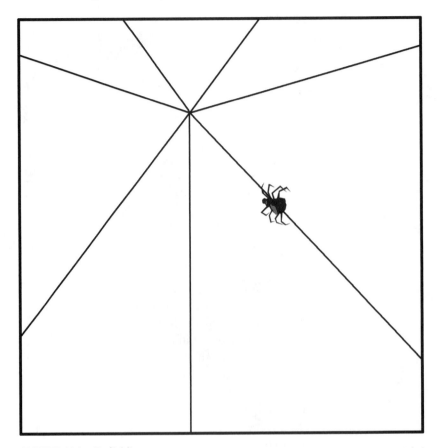

FIGURE 10.3   Radial lines.

We may accept the relationships life gives us as a simple fact, complete with all the rules and assumptions ascribed by our family and culture. Or we may explore them with an inner awareness that develops a dynamic and expansive connection between the given and the potential that resides on the edge. What constitutes your core relationships, and how might they be enhanced or expanded?

> Relationship with one's ancestry:
> >   Develop intergenerational awareness
> >   Practice conscious choices
> Relationship with one's core beliefs:
> >   Develop focused intent
> >   Practice mindful awareness
> Relationship with one's environment:
> >   Develop vibrant health

Practice flexible adaptation
Relationship with one's whole self:
    Develop emotional balance
    Practice authentic presence
Relationship with others:
    Develop meaningful connections
    Practice compassionate caring
Relationship with life's lessons:
    Develop meaning in the experience
    Practice community service

IV. Spiral lines—self-creating: Living organisms go through a sequence of structural changes over time. At any point the structure is a record of all previous exchanges. However, life is ongoing and dynamic, and the generation of new configurations is possible as awareness grows within the organism, enlarging its choices for response.

Spiderwoman begins the process of weaving the web through a series of experiences and experiments. She is guided by an instinct and awareness that grows as her capacity and maturity increase. Size and shape changes as she brings new materials to the structure of her initial web.

Humankind also engages with our self-made reality, expanding its edges and capacity through *ways of knowing,* which set the focal point of thought that guides our actions. See Figure 10.4.

We can take information and events at face value while sitting in the frozen core. Or we can expand our experiences, learning from them as we continue to enlarge our web of connections and consciousness through purposeful living. How do you seek, assimilate, and interpret information and experiences in your life?

Information: accumulation of facts:
    Seeing clearly
    Concrete analysis
Knowledge: your lived experience:
    Assimilating events
    Reflective practice
Wisdom: deep knowing of focused attention:
    Intuitive knowing
    Creative responding
Mystery: unknowable as inspiration:
    Reverence for life
    Recognizing All-That-Is

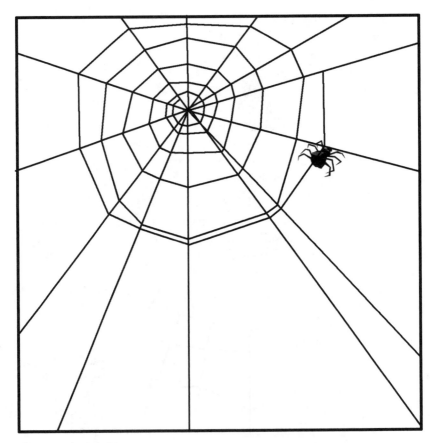

FIGURE 10.4   Spiral lines.

V. A healing web—self-renewing: Every living organism continually renews itself, breaking down and rebuilding structures while maintaining its overall identity. Organic systems are constantly exposed to hazard, so they have an innate ability to reproduce. While sexual reproduction is the origin of life, sharing resources in the form of community is the larger part of survival. Moving through cycles of give and take, a cell or a community find strength in reciprocity.

A healing web is part of a nested hierarchy; it is also part of a larger web of life. Life is a dynamic, richly textured, and ever-expanding network of connections, relationships, experiences, and reflective moments that enlarge our capacity while supporting Mother Earth and others in the ecosystem in their own web-work. See Figure 10.5.

By establishing and maintaining a dynamic web of connections and processes within one's life and to the larger universal web of life, holistic and sustainable existence will be possible for all.

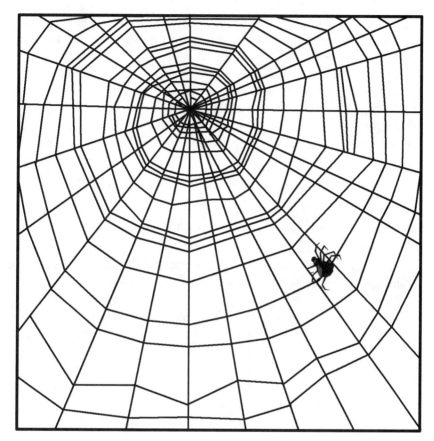

FIGURE 10.5   A healing web.

TRANSPERSONAL NURSING: BEING A HEALING PRESENCE

The privilege of being a nurse gives us multiple opportunities for expansive and cocreative relationships that enlarge our capacities and sensibilities. To partner with society in its quest for health deliberately and with compassion is the call for authentic nurses. These nurses know their own worldview while appreciating and drawing on the view of others. While they understand illness and institutional caring, they are equally at home in roles fostering health within every sector of society.

Noted quantum physicist Dana Zohar made a startling discovery (1990). After the birth of her daughter she became a mother. She then had a son and found that she was a different being. The role and responses in the relationship were decidedly different than the one shared with her daughter. She concluded that, like the elements in quantum physics, we are a quantum self. If we show up authentically and engage in the moment, we cocreate our reality with another, just as particles and waves cocreate the universe. The more true relationships we engage in, the more dimensions emerge in our personality and consciousness. There is no limit to the endless variations and iterations of self that reside in each of us if we remain an open system, hovering with flexibility on the edge of chaos.

The unconditional, transpersonal presence of a nurse creates an environment for healing. It is predicated on five principles of engagement for nursing.

1. Health and Well-Being Unfold Between One Nurse and One Patient in Each Authentic Encounter

The nursing profession has spent so much effort in the recent past to attain legitimacy within the health care industry that the authentic essence of nursing has been misplaced. In times of unprecedented change and chaos, such as a disruptive illness event, we demonstrate the natural tendency of reaching deeply to touch our own true roots. When nurses and patients establish a relationship based on respect and unconditional regard, a space opens for deep inner reflection and remembering. It is here that the seeds of potential for continuing growth and unfolding reside.

> *Authenticity* moves one to their true essence, inviting others to their own so all can celebrate the art of being human rather than the role of being perfect. Real is more life-giving than perfect or best.

- Speak and listen authentically
- See clearly
- Act spontaneously with the power of your intuition
- Be impeccable with the truth
- Practice gratitude and affirmation
- Extend grace and forgiveness

2. Reflective Practice Is the Hallmark of an Authentic Nurse

Nursing is a practice discipline of applied science. Nurses face challenging and unique situations that call for flexible ways of responding to and learning from the situation. Mezirow (1991) suggests that professionals are often faced with situations of uncertainty, instability, and complexity that are unique and insoluble by the strict application of scientific and technical knowledge. At the *center* of professional competence lies the capacity to learn how to learn. *A major tool that facilitates learning through practice is reflection.*

Reflective practice is a two stage process. *Reflection-in-action* occurs while practicing, which influences decisions made in the moment. *Reflection-on-action* occurs after the event, contributing to further development of practice skills and the creation of meaning.

– Identify a distorting dilemma as experienced
– Initiate the process of self-examination, recognizing it may contain feelings of guilt, shame, or confusion
– Perform a critical assessment of biological, social, cultural, religious, and psychic assumptions that you made
– Share the thoughts and ideas selectively with respected others
– Recognize that your discontent and assumptions are shared and that others have negotiated a similar situation, creating a sense of encouragement and community
– Explore options for new roles, relationships, and actions, with renewed courage from the examples of others transformational experiences
– Try new practice protocols or new roles provisionally
– Build competence and self-confidence as the experiment with alternatives leads to changing outcomes and increased comfort
– Reintegrate enlarging attitudes and behaviors into your life on the basis of conditions dictated by your new perspective

3. Authentic, Reflective Practice Enhances Potential for Intuition and Creativity

Authentic, reflective practitioners hold the capacity to engage meaningfully with multiple perspectives simultaneously. Surfing between lower and higher mind, their active intelligence, rather than the concrete mind, is the guiding light for discernment. This brings both inner wisdom and professional judgment to bear upon the situation.

Complex and unsettling circumstances prompt them to align all they know with what others know that has not been their lived experience. By starting with what is known and moving that knowledge into more abstract thought, adaptive clinical applications can be created. The nurse and the patient both develop an increasingly complex understanding of the phenomenon of healing in their shared world.

Enhanced intuition facilitates practical science; tapping into the repertoire of understanding from analysis and understanding of one's cumulative collection of patient experiences.

- Listen for the meaning behind the words in the patient's story
- Notice incongruence between spoken word and body language
- Sense the significant and important in the patient's experience
- Explore exaggerated reactions to unfolding events
- Note your body's messages as you provide specific care procedures
- Practice silence before speaking; let what is trying to emerge occur
- Pay attention to the subtle

4. Intuitive Practice Facilitates the Uncovering of Meaning in the Illness Event

Meaning is the way in which we use a life experience to grow and deepen as human beings. The creative and responsive nurse combines *quick knowledge*— a problem-solving approach accomplished through the nursing process—with aspects of *slower wisdom* – longitudinal examination of issues over time. Her capacity to weave facts and stories combines the art and science of nursing in a way that gives meaning to the experience for all parties involved.

Complexity confounds and confuses a situation. Balanced order and organization takes the complications out of complexity, allowing the meaning of the event to be discovered and honored. Authentic, reflective practitioners, armed with an innate understanding of the interdependence of all things, assist individuals, families, and communities in understanding the origin of the illness event. Together they cocreate protocols and programs that bring understanding and stability to the complexity in their lives on issues surrounding health.

Unfolding meaning emerges from *pattern recognition, which is the essence of integration.* A seven-generation viewpoint is essential to identifying family of origin, cultural, social, and ecological issues and their impact on the individual, family, and community.

- Be present in the moment
- Move into purposeful not-knowing
- Examine the issue by looking at its role in relationship to: family, organization, community, Mother Earth, seven generations out, and finally, oneself
- Ask intuitive versus curious questions

- Develop a playful attitude
- *Know* your own mind—the values and beliefs that guide, enhance, and limit your view so you do not project them onto others
- Recapture a child's sense of awe, wonder, and discovery

5. Compassion Creates the Context for Transpersonal Caring

Transpersonal care must be offered with a sense of humility and compassion as we realize that each life event plays a healthy role within a process far greater than the event itself. The whole idea of compassion is based on a keen awareness of the interdependence of all living beings, which are all part of one another and all involved in one another. As we cocreate a unified perspective we naturally move towards surrender to what is trying to emerge.

> *Compassion* requires us to connect with openness and softness of heart: being there for others without withdrawing. As we develop compassion for our own wounds, we move to unconditional compassion for ourselves, which naturally leads to compassion for others.
>
> - Recognize that compassion is an awareness you become rather than something you do
> - Allow things to simply be versus making and doing
> - Develop the capacity to make a judgment without judging
> - Foster choice-making for the patient; abuse is the absence of choice
> - Realize that to take responsibility for solving problems that belong to others is a misuse of your role and power
> - Develop the compassionate ability to simply bear witness, allowing others the outcome of their own experience

Compassion for others begins with kindness to oneself. It is very healing to stop hiding from ourselves. We can do this as we make friends with what we reject in ourselves. We are invited to be generous with what we cherish about ourselves. We suddenly realize that we already have everything we need. There is no need for self-improvement. Unwanted things in us awaken compassion for ourselves, and then for others. They show us how to work open-heartedly with life *just as it is.*

> We are losing our capacity to be human as violence and oppression are commonplace. We must grow towards compassion. The whole idea of

compassion is based on a keen awareness of the interdependence of all living beings, which are all part of one another, and all are involved in one another.

Thomas Merton

TRANSFORMING OURSELVES

Every part of scientific knowledge fits within the greater framework of our inner wisdom. We come to appreciate that each moment is unique, fresh, sacred, and it happens only once. And as we come to know and appreciate our deep connection with All-That-Is, we realize that we are not alone. We recognize that we are both the weaver and the web, the creator and the creation. Our attitudes and motivations flow from the wisdom of the soul.

As we move into wholeness we have developed ourselves fully. We are now secure in our selfless individuality. We become comfortable with selflessness, feeling more relaxed, energized, and joyful as we engage creatively with the world. Our gestures are meaningful and gracious, bringing a sense of the divine into our everyday lives. Universal good emanates from our compassionate acts of healing out into the world. Everything we say and do becomes a work of art.

A nurse whose essence emanates a healing presence offers the patient *hope*—oxygen for the soul. She or he believes in the goodness of human life, giving people insight to be and believe in the better part of themselves. She also demonstrates hope's twin, *courage*—the fuel that renews the energy of hope. Every new departure of human mind and spirit is an act of courage—arising from a life of authenticity.

Transformative nursing has an *enlarging vision* for the discipline—wings that will carry us to new realms of possibility. We will be lifted beyond rationality, propelled into a compassionate response to issues of the times. It also has *will* to follow through on this compelling vision with commitment and passion. The transpersonal healing presence of nursing is dedicated to shaping new order as an artist molds clay into an exquisite work of art. It is this sacred vehicle that will redefine nursing as a profession, ushering the discipline into the next millennium—with imagination, integrity, and grace.

> *For all sick beings in the world*
> *May I be the doctor and the medicine,*
> *And may I be the nurse*
> *Until every single one is healed!*

May a rain of food and drink descend on all
To clear away the pain of thirst and hunger,
And during the great eon of famine
May I turn myself into food and drink!
May I become an inexhaustible treasure
For those who are poor and destitute;
May I turn into all the things they could need,
And may these be placed close beside them!
Just like a blind man who discovers
A precious jewel in a trash heap,
By some good fortune I have found
The enlightening soul within me!
This is the ultimate medicine
That cures all the world's diseases
The tree that shades all beings who roam
Sadly on the road of terminal lives!

Excerpts from the Bodhisattva Vow

BIBLIOGRAPHY

Bunkers, S., Brentro, M., Johnson, S., Koerner, J., Larson, J., Karpiuk, K., et al. (1992, February). The healing web: A transformative model for nursing. *Nursing and Healthcare, 13*(2), 68–73.

Capra, F. (1996). *The web of life: A new scientific understanding of living systems.* New York: Anchor Books Doubleday.

Kauffman, S. (1993). *The origins of order.* New York: Oxford University Press.

Larson, J., Koerner, J., Bunkers, S., Brentron, M., Johnson, S., Karpiuk, K., et al. (1993, May). The healing web: A transformative model for nursing part II. *Nursing and Healthcare, 13*(5), 246–252.

Mezirow, J. (1991). *Transformative dimensions of adult learning.* San Francisco: Jossey-Bass.

Pilisuk, M., & Parks, S. H. (1989). *The healing web: Social networks and human survival.* Boston: University Press of New England.

Zohar, D. (1990). *The quantum self: Human nature and consciousness defined by the new physics.* New York: William Morrow.

Afterword

Encouragement for Your Journey

Withdraw into your self and look.
And if you do not find yourself beautiful yet,
do as does the creator of a statue that is to be
made beautiful; he cuts away here, there,
he makes this line lighter, this other purer, until
he has shown a beautiful face upon his statue.
So do you also; cut away all that is excessive,
straighten all that is crooked, bring to light all
that is shadow, labor to make all glow with beauty,
and do not cease chiseling your statue until
there shall shine out on you the godlike splendour
of virtue, until you shall see the final goodness
surely established in the stainless shrine.
And when you have made this perfect work...
call up all your confidence strike forward
yet a step—you need a guide no longer.

Plotinus

Glossary of Terms

Active: An awareness coming from a place beyond the thinking mind

- *Active intelligence*—moving beyond the concrete thought of logic, analysis, and understanding to an active stance of knowing that incorporates intuition, intent, and inner wisdom
- *Active observation*—moving from passive looking to an active stance of observation by assessing both the concrete body and the subtle, while entering the nurse-patient experience from the perspective of relationship rather than an interventional viewpoint
- *Active receptivity*—the feminine function, an active principle of wholeness, a figure-ground dynamism that exposes the invisible half, which gives context and meaning to that which it gently uplifts and holds

Aspects of nursing: domains, focus, and roles of practice

- *Nursing science*—realm of concrete thought; the *evaluator aspect* of the role, focusing on observable and measurable facts, data, logic to guide evidence-based practice
- *Nursing art*—realm of abstract thought; the *interpreter aspect* of the role, guided by intuition and active awareness, which recognizes pattern and meaning
- *Nursing essence*—realm of healing presence; the *witness aspect* of the role, guided by no-thought, which creates a space of active receptivity that potentiates healing

Dinergy: the creative energy of organic growth

Essence of the divine—the highest manifestation of being a human can express

- *Divine spark*—the core self, a direct extension of the Source, the highest vibrational energy spectrum of humankind
- *Spiritual ego*—creates the region of the abstract world at three levels:

- *Will*—the intent behind the creative impulse, which calls forth a germinal idea and begins to move it towards manifestation
- *Wisdom*—pure, focused attention, which links us to intuition, which is the inner wisdom of primordial intelligence; the quintessence of all our previous life experiences
- *Active intelligence*—the upper sphere of the thought world, which serves as the gateway into the abstract world. When contacted through simple awareness, a shift in the focal point from concrete to abstract thought occurs, engaging our intuition and inner wisdom.
- *Soul-essence of being*—home of personal divinity, our unique capacities and life destiny. It is also home of inner wisdom and conscience, which gives direction and meaning to our life.

Force-matter: coalescing energy that is turning into form

Human energy fields: the multidimensional human organism

- *Gross physical body*—coarsest level, inert mineral machine
- *Vital etheric body*—energy wrapper that provides the structural and functional blueprints for the forms and programs of organic structures in the body
- *Desire-emotional body*—expresses desires, urges, emotions, and higher aspirations
- *Mental-reflective body*—reflects the body of thought, knowledge, and experience
- *Causal body*—outer sheath of body-mind-spirit that houses the spiritual ego

Levels of reality: our level of consciousness determines reality; increasing awareness creates a more intricate nervous system capable of environmental interaction in a more complex pattern.

- *Consensual reality*—shared perception of things that can be seen or touched, which are validated by the science and culture of the times
- *Inner reality*—highly individualized perception of inner experiences of fantasies, subjective feelings, emotions, and dreams
- *Core essence*—a highly developed perception of the subtle energy field behind the form being observed

Prana: vital life force a form of universal energy, originating from the sun, which is transformed into vitality globules in the spleen to energetically nourish the physical body

Real power: the ability to create our own reality, to live our own life, and to fulfill our destiny. This occurs when we effectively manage both "fast" and "slow" feelings.

- *Fast feelings*—spurred by fear or aggression create swift and decisive movement as they are part of our survival mechanism, housed in the reptilian and mammalian portions of our brain and concrete thought
- *Slow feelings*—such as stillness and complex memories foster nonaction, are essential for the unfolding of human potential, and are housed in out-of-body consciousness

Seed atoms: crystal forms of spiritual anatomy that contain all attributes and knowledge acquired through all evolutions of the consciousness cycles and stored in the causal body

- *Seed atom of physical body*—located in left ventricle of the heart, captures holographic pictures of all life events
- *Seed atom of vital body*—located in solar plexus, captures all modifications made to vital blueprints in this lifetime
- *Seed atom of desire-body*—located in the liver, records all emotional thoughts and urges as well as higher aspirations
- *Seed atom of concrete mind*—located in frontal sinus, records all thoughts, ideas, and creative ventures within the current life journey
- *Silver cord*—joins four seed atoms of the personality, connecting all our bodies of consciousness

Shifting the focal point: moving the focus of attention from the lower world of concrete thought to the higher world of abstract thought

- *Region of concrete thought*—three lower levels of embodied thought manifest in the gross physical body as senses (vital etheric), feelings (desire emotional) and analysis and logic (lower portion of mental reflective)
- *Region of abstract thought*—the three higher levels of spiritual consciousness, which include wisdom (focused intuition), intent (will power), and our core *self* (divine spark of life)
- *Mid-level (fourth) of thought world*—region of archetypal forces, the place where thought crystallizes into form, the home of the focal point, whose location is determined by the vibratory level of the person
- *Mental mind-body*—an organized cloud of force-matter specialized from the region of concrete thought; vibrating at two levels, it serves as the bridge between the regions of concrete and abstract thought.

- *Concrete thought*—the lower vibrational sector, which serves as our vehicle for thinking, the 'i' of thought, emotion, personality, and ego
- *Abstract thought*—the higher vibrational sector, which serves as the seat of the intuitive mind and "I' of the higher intellect, the spiritual ego, and the portal for creative, germinal ideas that flow from the field of infinite possibility
- *Home of the soul*—our individuality and conscience, found in the sixth dimension over the heart chakra
- *Intuition*—the inner wisdom, located in the soul, that increasingly contributes aspects of our unique potential and provides guidance for us to move down the true path of our identity and destiny

Spheres of consciousness: human energy physiology includes consciousness at various stages of expression in each human being.

- *Objective universe*—essence of body—the concrete world of form: body, personality, and ego
- *Subjective universe*—essence of divine—the abstract spiritual world of being: spiritual ego and core *self*
- *Intermediate sphere*—essence of mind—the intermediate mental world of thought; functions as the focal point between concrete and abstract mind
- *Causal body*—vehicle of consciousness—the outer sheath covering body-mind-spirit; repository of essence of all previous lifetimes, home of spiritual ego

Spirit of Universal Consciousness: the universal spirit that is the deepest and most inclusive ground of being. Spirit is the source of all that exists. Spirit is the infinite, creative energy that gives birth to the universe. Spirit is the common source of the world's faith traditions. Spirit is the love that creates and sustains life.

Vision: the act of seeing

- *Passive mechanism*—ordinary sight or physical vision using organs of sight
- *Active mechanism*—perceptive mental vision using a radar-like system

Vitality globules: etheric corpuscles that provide energy nourishment for the body through force openings (chakras) located in vital etheric body

Index